David Elkins's new book is an enormous contribution to the fields of clinical psychology, counseling, psychotherapy, and related helping professions. It is one of the most persuasive treatises I have read on the shortcomings of the medical model of psychotherapy and the need for alternative approaches within the helping professions. Well reasoned, well written, and supported by considerable data, *Humanistic Psychology: A Clinical Manifesto* should be required reading for all graduate students in psychology, counseling, social work, pastoral psychology, nursing, and related fields.

Howard Kirschenbaum, EdD
Professor Emeritus, University of Rochester
Author, *The Life and Work of Carl Rogers* (2009)

+++++++

In clear, exact, and unrelenting terms, Dr. David Elkins diagnoses the disease ailing professional practice and proposes the cure. A "must read" for any professional hoping to survive the brave new world of clinical practice.

Scott D. Miller, PhD
International Centre for Clinical Excellence
(www.centerforclinicalexcellence.com),
Co-editor of *The Heart and Soul of Change: What Works in Psychotherapy*

++++++

Dave Elkins's wonderful new book carries forward the vision of psychotherapy of Carl Rogers and other humanistic psychologists. Elkins provides cogent criticisms of the medical model and mounts an inspired argument for a "human" psychotherapy that focuses on the power of the relationship and on working with clients to promote their own self-generated growth in contrast to current approaches which "do to" clients with technological interventions. A vision for the 21st century!

Arthur Bohart, PhD
Professor Emeritus, California State University Dominguez Hills
Faculty, Saybrook Graduate School
Co-author, *How Clients Make Therapy Work: The Process of Active Self Healing* Co-editor, *Empathy Reconsidered*

++++++

In a way, all scientific publications are rhetorical devices, hoping to use evidence to promote a particular conclusion. In that regard *Humanistic Psychology: A Clinical Manifesto* makes no bones about it—it is a manifesto. Elkins's intention is to create a revolution against the medicalization of psychotherapy and thereby reclaim the humanistic aspects of psychotherapy. But this is not a "soft headed" plea by a humanist—Elkins marshals the best available evidence to support the case that humanistic aspects of psychotherapy are absolutely essential components of effective psychotherapy. Along the way, he passionately builds the case for empathy, warmth, and compassion by providing a thorough review of the scientific literature situated in a rich, but largely forgotten, historical context. This is a volume that will change hearts and minds—it appeals to both, in a beautiful blend.

Bruce E. Wampold, PhD, ABPP,
Professor and Chair of the Department of Counseling Psychology and
Clinical Professor of Psychiatry, University of Wisconsin –Madison;
Author, *The Great Psychotherapy Debate: Models, Methods, and Findings;*
The Basics of Psychotherapy: An Introduction to Theory; and
The Heart and Soul of Change: Delivering What Works (2nd ed.)

++++++

Dr. Elkins is right: Clinical psychology as a profession has betrayed its humanistic and ethical roots in favor of the more remunerative and authoritarian medical model. Meanwhile, many individual psychologists feel alone and despairing over the moral and scientific collapse of their leadership. Dr. Elkins's book provides these psychologists with much-needed information and inspiration.

Peter R. Breggin, MD, psychiatrist
Author, *Medication Madness; Brain-Disabling Treatments in Psychiatry*;
The Heart of Being Helpful; and *Toxic Psychiatry.*

++++++

This book reveals the real inside story on the new therapy outcome research—humanistic psychology is back! With masterful strokes of both clarity and cogency, Elkins ignites the sparks of a truth that can no longer be ignored: The key to effective therapy is depth of connection, and the key to depth of connection is humanism.

Kirk J. Schneider, PhD
Editor of the *Journal of Humanistic Psychology*
Author, *Existential-Integrative Psychotherapy* and
Awakening to Awe: Personal Stories of Profound Transformation.

++++++

Manifesto indeed! 21st century psychologists need this book now more than ever as the conflict intensifies between reductionistic, dehumanizing therapies and those that honor whole persons. After 50 years of practice, I welcome Dave Elkins's book and wish I had it much earlier. It is essential reading for existential-humanistic clinicians, and indeed for all our colleagues who wish to keep up-to-date.

Thomas Greening, PhD
Professor of Psychology, Saybrook Graduate School,
International Editor of *Journal of Humanistic Psychology*

++++++

In this cry from the heart, David Elkins traces the path by which the creative aspirations that once made psychotherapy a powerful force for individual and social transformation became stifled, co-opted, and corporatized. As calls for health care reform get louder, the emancipatory principles at the center of a person-centered humanistic psychology offer some real and tested alternatives to therapist-centered service. Graduate students in all the mental health fields should read this book.

Maureen O'Hara, PhD
Professor of Psychology, National University,
President Emerita, Saybrook Graduate School,
Co-author, *10 Things to Do In A Conceptual Emergency*

++++++

If you are puzzled and concerned about the forces that undermine the impact of humanistic psychology and psychotherapy in an increasingly technological and inhumane world, then read this book. In a series of clear and well argued chapters, David Elkins takes on the limitations and failures of the medical model, the myth of Empirically Supported Treatments (ESTs), politics in graduate training, and psychology's loss of its heart and soul. Dr. Elkin's message is one of inspiration and hope. After reading this text, I felt energized and encouraged to renew my efforts to advance the fundamental perspectives and values of humanistic psychology.

David J. Cain, PhD
ABPP, Editor
Editor with Jules Seeman, of
Humanistic Psychotherapies: Handbook of Research and Practice
Author of forthcoming *Person-Centered Psychotherapies*

Humanistic Psychology: A Clinical Manifesto

A Critique of Clinical Psychology and the Need for Progressive Alternatives

David N. Elkins, PhD

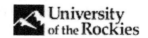

University of the Rockies Press
555 E. Pikes Peak Avenue, #108
Colorado Springs, Colorado 80903

First Published in 2009, University of the Rockies Press.

ISBN-10:	0-9764638-8-1
ISBN-13:	978-0-9764638-8-7

University of the Rockies Press
555 E. Pikes Peak Avenue, #108
Colorado Springs, CO 80903

Cover Design by Laura Ross, 2009

Chapter 1, "Whatever Happened to Carl Rogers? An Examination of the Politics of Clinical Psychology," copyright 2008 by David N. Elkins.

Chapter 2, "Short-Term, Linear Approaches to Psychotherapy: What We Now Know," is based on the following article: Elkins, D. N., *Journal of Humanistic Psychology, 48*(3) 413-43, copyright 2008 by Sage Publications, Inc. Reprinted by Permission of Sage Publications, Inc. Also, see SAGE Journals Online: http://online.sagepub.com.

Chapter 3, "The Medical Model in Psychotherapy: Its Limitations and Failures," is based on the following article: Elkins, D. N., *Journal of Humanistic Psychology, 49*(1), 66-84, copyright 2009 by Sage Publications, Inc. Reprinted by Permission of Sage Publications, Inc. Also, see SAGE Journals Online: http://online.sagepub.com

Chapter 4, "Empirically Supported Treatments: The Deconstruction of a Myth," is based on the following article: Elkins, D. N., *Journal of Humanistic Psychology, 47*(4), 474-500, copyright 2007 by Sage Publications, Inc. Reprinted by Permission of Sage Publications, Inc. Also, see SAGE Journals Online: http://online.sagepub.com

DEDICATION

PROFESSIONAL

To the Memory of Carl Rogers (1902-1987)

Nominee for the Nobel Peace Prize and the most influential clinical psychologist of the 20th century. His life and writings changed our lives by his gentle insistence that the power of transformation lay within ourselves.

PERSONAL

To David and Jody Elkins
Two sons with strong spirits and tender hearts.
What more could a father want?

Contents

Acknowledgements

This book might never have been written if it had not been for Louis Hoffman, editor-in-chief of University of the Rockies Press. After reading some articles I had written, Louis invited me to submit a proposal for what became this book. Thus, I owe a debt of gratitude to Louis for his initial encouragement and for his continuing support as the book developed.

I am also grateful to Natalie Rogers for her enthusiastic endorsement of the chapter on Carl Rogers, her father. Because Carl Rogers had such a powerful impact on my personal and professional life, I was deeply touched by Natalie's support of the book. She not only agreed to write the foreword but also offered insightful suggestions that made the book stronger.

I also thank Kirk Schneider, editor of the *Journal of Humanistic Psychology (JHP)* and Larry Leitner, former editor of *The Humanistic Psychologist (THP),* for publishing the original articles from which this book grew.

I thank Tom Greening, Maureen O'Hara, and Arthur Bohart who made helpful suggestions regarding the article that became Chapter Five of this book. I am responsible, of course, for any limitations of the chapter and for its point of view.

I am grateful to Bruce Wampold, Chair of the Department of Counseling Psychology and Professor of Psychiatry at the University of Wisconsin-Madison, for his ground-breaking research on contextual factors as the primary determinants of therapeutic effectiveness. Chapter Four of this book, which critiques so-called "empirically supported treatments," would not have been possible without his work. I also thank him for taking the time to clarify and elaborate on some of his findings when I was writing the original article on which Chapter Four is based. Again, I am responsible for any limitations of the chapter.

I thank Negar Shekarabi, my doctoral student and graduate assistant at Pepperdine University, for locating publications and performing other clerical duties at the time some of the original articles were being written. Negar is now Dr. Shekarabi, having received her PsyD degree in 2008.

I am also grateful to all my doctoral students in the Graduate School of Education and Psychology at Pepperdine University. Their bright, creative minds, along with their passionate desire for more humane perspectives in clinical psychology, gave me the courage to criticize my profession and to put in writing the values and perspectives articulated in this book. This is the great secret of academia: professors always learn more from their students than their students learn from them.

I also thank Laura Ross, a woman with an excellent artistic sense, who designed the cover for the book.

I thank Trent Claypool, Jason Dias, and Michael Moats for assisting with the preparation of the index and editorial work.

I am grateful to Sara, my wife and "editor-in-residence," whose unerring sense of good, efficient writing forced me to delete from this book some of the finest-sounding superfluities I had ever written. I am also grateful to Jody and Sandy Elkins, our son and daughter-in-law, who enthusiastically supported the project and helped choose the final cover design.

Finally, I am grateful to Sage Publications, publisher of the *Journal of Humanistic Psychology*, and Routledge, Taylor & Francis Group, publisher of *The Humanistic Psychologist*, for granting me permission to use articles that were originally published in those journals.

Editor's Preface

My first contact with David Elkins was little more than a year ago when I asked him to write a few lines for the book cover of Tom Greening's book, *Words Against the Void: Poems by an Existential Psychologist.* When I received what Dave wrote, my immediate reaction was that this was not only an endorsement but a contribution to the book; it placed the book and its purpose in context while providing a frame of reference for how the book should be read. The combination of insight along with the poetic quality of his writing intrigued me.

For many years I had been familiar with Dave's writing and contributions. However, around this time a flurry of recent articles by Dave in the *Journal of Humanistic Psychology* was beginning to create a buzz in humanistic and existential circles. As I read the articles, I immediately recognized that these were some of the most important contributions to humanistic psychology in many years. With striking insight, Dave approached controversial topics, such as the empirically supported treatments movement, the medical model, and the discounting and minimizing of humanistic psychology's contribution. Most of the other responses I read on these topics were either defensive or did not reflect an awareness of the breadth of literature on the topics. In contrast, Dave addressed the most important and pressing issues for humanistic psychology with full awareness of the various perspectives on these issues in humanistic psychology and beyond.

At the same time, the University of the Rockies Press was searching for important manuscripts on existential and humanistic psychology. It was clear to me that there was no more needed contribution than what Dave's writing had been addressing. When I contacted him to ask if he would be interested in turning the ideas in his articles into a book, I was certain someone must have already asked him to do this. I was pleasantly surprised when this was not the case and he agreed to put together a proposal for our press.

Humanistic Psychology: A Clinical Manifesto is not only about the present state of affairs in humanistic psychology, but it is also a book about what the future of the discipline ought to be. The book is not overly idealistic, nor is it burdened by the pessimistic view that humanistic psychology has moved on from its "glory days." Instead, the book is honest about where things are and reflects a passionate perspective about the direction we should go. Borrowing from the words of Kevin Keenan, this book is about "the futuring of humanistic psychology."

As I read through the final manuscript, I was again reminded of the importance and timeliness of this book. I am convinced that, more than any other manuscript I have ever read, this has the potential to be a book that could change the face of humanistic psychology and maybe even impact mainstream psychology. It is a book that needed to be written and there is no one better to have written it than Dave.

Louis Hoffman, PhD
Editor-in-Chief, University of the Rockies Press
Co-Editor, *Existential Psychology East-West*

Foreword

A few months ago David Elkins sent me an article that he had written about my father's work titled "Whatever Happened to Carl Rogers? An Examination of the Politics of Clinical Psychology." (The article is now Chapter One of this book). As I read the manuscript, I found myself saying, "Bravo!" and "Yes!" and "Thank you!" I sent David an e-mail saying, among other things, that I agreed with his view that the medical model in academic clinical psychology is well-entrenched and still resisting Carl's discoveries about the importance of personal and interpersonal factors in psychotherapy. From the time Carl first wrote about his client-centered approach, he encountered strong opposition from those who believed the therapist should be "in charge" and "administer treatments" to the "patient." Even Carl's extensive research during his tenure at the University of Chicago did not stop the critics, even though that research consistently showed that relational factors – not techniques – were the major ingredients of therapeutic effectiveness. It says something about the power of the medical model in American psychology that Carl's discoveries are so often ignored or marginalized today. I find it encouraging, however, that contemporary research has confirmed (once again) that personal and interpersonal factors are at the center of therapeutic healing. I share David's hope that these scientific findings will create a revolution that dethrones, once and for all, the medical model in psychotherapy and establishes in its place a more relational and scientifically grounded approach to counseling and psychotherapy.

If that revolution comes about, I believe *Humanistic Psychology: A Clinical Manifesto* will be considered as one of the books that helped ignite it. In this well-documented and highly readable book, David examines the politics of clinical psychology. In that process he skillfully dismantles major myths of clinical psychology and summarizes recent research that undermines the medical model. The book is indeed a "clinical manifesto" and one that is long overdue. I highly recommend this book and believe it will enjoy a wide readership. It is the kind of book that my father, Carl Rogers, would have enthusiastically endorsed.

Natalie Rogers, PhD
Author of *Emerging Woman* and *The Creative Connection:*
Expressive Arts as Healing
Distinguished Consulting Faculty
Saybrook Graduate School
www.nrogers.com

I called the book a "clinical manifesto" because I wanted to make it clear that the book is not only a scholarly work but also a political statement, a formal proclamation of humanistic values and perspectives that challenges the entrenched medical model ideology of mainstream clinical psychology.

Introduction

I am launching this book at the dawn of what may be the greatest revolution in the history of psychotherapy. The essence of that revolution is that the medical model, which dominated clinical psychology for more than 100 years, has been scientifically discredited, and clinical psychology must now create a new paradigm to account for therapeutic effectiveness and to guide training and practice. The revolution was created by recent research--in the form of analyses and meta-analyses of thousands of psychotherapy studies --which makes it clear that modalities and techniques have little to do with therapeutic effectiveness and that "contextual factors" are the major determinants of therapeutic outcome. (See Chapter Four for extensive documentation of this statement). These findings are a devastating blow to the medical model. They undermine the basic assumptions of the model and leave the field of clinical psychology in disarray, creating an urgent need for a new paradigm of training and practice that will reflect and incorporate these findings.

Most clinical psychologists are unaware that the world has shifted and that the old paradigm is now obsolete. As a result, the vast majority of our clinics, training programs, and research centers still embrace the medical model, making it seem that the model is alive and well. But increasing numbers of clinicians and scholars are reading the research on contextual factors and realizing its radical implications for the future of psychotherapy. I am hopeful that those numbers will soon reach critical mass, forcing the power sectors of clinical psychology to acknowledge the death of the medical model and to begin creating a new model of practice and training that emphasizes contextual factors and reflects the latest scientific research.

I wrote this book for several reasons: First, I wrote it because it is now clear that clinical psychology is in trouble. Clinical psychology has a cancer and the name of that cancer is the medical model. The cancer has spread to our clinics, training programs, internships, and research centers. The cancer permeates our language, articles, and books. It has spread to the American Psychological Association (APA) so that publications of our national organization now read like medical literature. With no sense of metaphor, we speak of "diagnosing" the "pathology" of "patients" and "administering treatments" to "cure" "mental disorders." In our training programs, we indoctrinate students in medical model ideology, turning them into "junior physicians" who must think and talk in medical model jargon in order to graduate and receive our blessings. Contemporary clinical psychology is so permeated by the medical model, so entangled with it politically and economically, that it is almost impossible to remove the cancer without killing the profession. Yet, the surgery is necessary because the scientific research has now made it clear that the medical model is wrong and if we continue to support this discredited model, we will find ourselves on the opposite side of science with no place to stand when the foundations begin to shake.

Second, I wrote the book because I believe it is time for humanistic psychologists to speak out. I called the book a "clinical manifesto" because I wanted to make it clear that the book is not only a scholarly work but also a political statement, a formal proclamation of humanistic values and perspectives that challenges the entrenched medical model ideology of mainstream clinical psychology. For nearly 70 years, beginning with Carl Rogers in the 1940s, humanistic psychologists have insisted that the medical model is problematic and that personal and interpersonal factors--not medical-like techniques-- are at the center of therapeutic healing. During most of those years, mainstream clinical psychology insisted that the medical model was right and poured millions of dollars into thousands of efficacy studies in search of specific techniques for specific disorders. Generally speaking, that effort has been a failure. In fact, when one considers the amount of money and time involved, that research effort was probably the biggest boondoggle in the history of psychotherapy research. Ironically, many of those efficacy studies were included in the recent meta-analytic studies which determined that "contextual factors"--not modalities or techniques--were the major determinants of therapeutic effectiveness! Contextual factors, which are found in all therapeutic approaches, include such elements as the alliance, the relationship, the qualities of the therapist, client agency, allegiance, client expectations, and extra-therapeutic factors. Although the term includes more than the personal and interpersonal elements of therapy, it is nevertheless true that personal and interpersonal elements are major determinants of therapeutic outcome while techniques have little to do with therapeutic effectiveness. *Thus, humanistic psychology was right and mainstream clinical psychology was wrong*. This is a powerful vindication of humanistic psychology-- a vindication that is still generally unacknowledged by the mainstream. Nevertheless, this puts humanistic scholars in a unique position to make significant contributions to the future of psychotherapy. Humanistic psychology has a rich literature on the therapeutic relationship and on how to facilitate the personal and interpersonal growth of both clients and therapist trainees. Thus, it is time for humanistic psychologists to speak up and to offer new directions to a profession that went down the wrong road.

Third, I wrote the book because "medical model" psychologists are not the only therapists out there. Thousands of counseling psychologists, marriage and family therapists, multicultural therapists, feminist therapists, constructivist therapists, humanistic therapists, existential therapists, transpersonal therapists, pastoral counselors, clinical social workers, and even some psychiatrists and clinical psychologists eschew the medical model and know that it does not accurately describe what actually occurs in psychotherapy. Many therapists are frustrated that psychology has betrayed its own identity and donned the ill-fitting garb of the medical profession. They know from their own experience that psychotherapy is an interpersonal process, not a medical procedure, and they have no desire to be "junior physicians." I wrote this book to encourage such professionals and to support their efforts to conceptualize and structure their clinical work in alternative ways.

Fourth, I wrote the book for students. For more than 20 years I taught in a traditional psychology program where I helped to train clinical psychologists. As a professor, I watched beginning students-- full of passion and idealism--slowly wilt under the burdensome ideology of the medical model and the type of training that accompanies it. Most students enter training because they want to dedicate their lives to helping those who are suffering from emotional pain. Many have been told by family and friends that their warm, compassionate nature makes them "naturals" when it comes to counseling and psychotherapy. But something happens on the way to becoming a clinical psychologist. To their dismay and consternation, students discover that many of their professors and supervisors are not impressed by their compassionate attitudes and interpersonal abilities. They are told, implicitly or explicitly, that in order to become a "real psychologist" they must learn to think in medical model terms and learn medical model techniques and procedures. Oh yes, empathy and compassion are all fine and good but only as ways to "soften up" clients so that they will be more cooperative and compliant with the "treatment." Eager to learn and wanting to please, most students throw themselves into their graduate work. They abandon their natural instincts to learn a system that feels alien but which, everyone seems to agree, is the only way to become a clinical psychologist. By the end of their doctoral training, most students have been transformed into medical-like experts who "diagnose" "pathology" and "administer treatments" to "cure" "mental disorders." They have become "junior physicians."

And what about empathy, warmth, and compassion? Does clinical training help students cultivate such personal and interpersonal qualities? Generally speaking, the answer is no. Peter Breggin (1991), a psychiatrist, said, "Nowhere in my formal psychiatric training was there a serious discussion of caring, compassion, or love" (P. Breggin, personal communication, August 27, 2009.). Most clinical psychologists would have to say the same about their training. This shows how far we have strayed from what matters. Purportedly, clinical psychology is dedicated to the alleviation of emotional suffering, yet in clinical training one almost never hears anything about caring, compassion, or love. Why is this true? Because the medical model, which dominates contemporary clinical training, focuses on "techniques" and one does not have to be a warm, compassionate human being in order to "administer techniques" any more than a brain surgeon has to be a warm, compassionate human being in order to do brain surgery. In other words, the medical model militates against the personal and interpersonal development of therapists because the model assumes that *techniques* are responsible for healing the client, not the personal and interpersonal qualities of the therapist. But because science has now shown that techniques have little to do with therapeutic effectiveness while the personal and interpersonal dimensions of therapy are major determinants of therapeutic outcome, it is time for clinical training programs, if they wish to produce highly effective therapists, to reduce the emphasis on specific modalities and techniques and emphasize, instead, the personal and interpersonal development of students. The new goal of clinical training should be to produce caring, compassionate, and deeply human therapists instead of "junior physicians" with a bag of techniques.

Finally, it is not enough simply to criticize. If humanistic psychologists are to make significant contributions to the future of clinical psychology, we must work with others to create a new model of training and practice. In that regard, I am already planning a companion volume that will provide a positive vision of what training and practice might "look like" if the medical model were eliminated and the contextual factors were placed at center stage. Therefore, as you read this book, which presents a rather intense critique of contemporary clinical psychology, please think of it as "clearing the ground" so that a new model of training and practice--something more compassionate and humane--might have a place to grow.

*I am not suggesting that Rogers's ideas should
dominate clinical training. I am merely suggesting
that they should be **included** and given their proper
due. The fact that they are not raises serious
questions about the politics of clinical training in
America*

Chapter One

Whatever Happened to Carl Rogers?
An Examination of the Politics of Clinical Psychology

Chapter Overview*: The chapter examines why Carl Rogers, one of
the most important clinicians in history, is often ignored by
contemporary clinical psychology. The chapter sets the tone for the
book and provides a concrete example of how political forces shape
clinical training and practice.*

Contemporary clinical psychology doesn't quite know what to
do with Carl Rogers. On the one hand, it is widely acknowledged that
Rogers changed the landscape of American psychology. Rogers
authored 16 books, published more than 200 scholarly articles, gave
hundreds of professional presentations, and engaged in public
dialogues with some of the most influential thinkers of his era
including Martin Buber and Paul Tillich (Kirschenbaum, 2009;
Kirschenbaum & Henderson, 1989; N. Rogers, 2008). Rogers's
theories have had an impact on education, social work, nursing,
counseling, psychotherapy, group therapy, peace efforts, and
interpersonal relations. His theories have generated more research
than those of any other clinical psychologist in American history
(Bozarth, Zimring, & Tausch, 2001; Kirschenbaum, 2009). Rogers
and his contributions are recognized internationally, and he received
awards and honorary degrees from dozens of groups, organizations,
and institutions at home and abroad. The American Psychological
Association (APA) gave Rogers two of its most prestigious awards--
the "Award for Distinguished Scientific Contributions" in 1956 and
the "Award for Distinguished Professional Contributions to

Psychology" in 1972. He was the first psychologist in history to receive both awards (Cain, 2001a). In a 1982 survey of psychologists conducted by the *American Psychologist* (see D. Smith, 1982), Rogers was named as the most influential psychotherapist and 25 years later, in a survey conducted by the *Psychotherapy Networker* (April/March, 2007), Rogers was again ranked number one. Also, in a study by Haggbloom et al. (2002) that ranked the 100 most eminent psychologists of the twentieth century based on multiple criteria that included professional psychology journal citations, introductory psychology textbook citations, and survey responses from members of the American Psychological Society, Rogers received an overall ranking of six and for clinicians he was second only to Sigmund Freud. In his later years Rogers conducted group workshops in Northern Ireland and South Africa in an effort to promote communication and understanding. For these efforts, he was nominated for the Nobel Peace Prize in 1987 (Cain, 2001a).

It would be difficult to overestimate the significance of Rogers's contributions to clinical psychology. Often called the "father of psychotherapy research," he was the first to record and analyze the transcripts of actual therapy sessions in an effort to clarify what makes for effective psychotherapy; he was the first clinician to conduct major studies on psychotherapy using quantitative methods; he was the first to formulate a comprehensive theory of personality and psychotherapy grounded in quantitative research; he was the first to develop a theory of psychotherapy that de-emphasized pathology and that focused, instead, on the strengths and potentials of clients (Bozarth, Zimring, & Tausch, 2001; Cain, 2001a; Rogers, 1957). Today, Rogers's ideas are echoed every time psychologists talk about the importance of the therapeutic relationship, raise concerns about the medical model, discuss the significance of the personal qualities of the therapist, or mention the importance of contextual factors in therapeutic outcome (see Wampold, 2001). Even Seligman's "Positive Psychology," a contemporary movement that has attracted hundreds of psychologists, is little more than a reframing of Rogers's original emphasis on the strengths and potentials of clients (see Elkins, 2009b; Greening & Bohart, 2001; Resnick, Warmoth, & Serlin, 2001; Seligman & Csikszentmihalyi, 2000).

The Question Addressed in This Chapter

In light of his many contributions, one would think that a large number of contemporary clinical psychologists would embrace client-centered perspectives and that Rogers and his ideas would be an important part of all training programs in clinical psychology. This, however, is not the case. The truth is, only 10% of clinical psychologists identify themselves as "humanistic" and client-centered therapists are a subset of that group (Cain, 2001b). Further, many training programs in clinical psychology marginalize or ignore Rogers and his contributions (see Cain, 2001b; Elkins, 2007; Wertz, 1998). For example, as a professor in a post-masters doctoral program, I found that most incoming doctoral students were unfamiliar with the research on client-centered therapy, could not articulate Rogers's theory of personality, and were not even aware that he had a developmental theory. Even more disturbing, many clinical professors know little about Rogers and often hold stereotypical and misinformed views about his contributions (see Chapter Five or Elkins, 2009b). Clearly, something is wrong when one of the most important clinicians in history is ignored in clinical training. Keep in mind that I am not suggesting that Rogers's ideas should *dominate* clinical training. I am merely suggesting that they should be *included* and given their proper due. The fact that they are not raises serious questions about the politics of clinical training in America.

Thus, the question addressed in this chapter is: *Why do so many contemporary clinical psychologists and training programs in clinical psychology marginalize or ignore Rogers and his ideas?* I realize that some would answer this question by saying that Rogers is now out of date or that any substantial contributions he made have already been incorporated into clinical psychology. I would suggest, however, that such answers represent further dismissals of Rogers--the very problem this chapter addresses--and reveal a serious failure to grasp the nature and extent of his contributions. *Thus, in this chapter I will suggest a very different answer as to why Rogers is ignored--one based on an examination of the politics of clinical psychology.*

Carl Rogers and the Psychiatric Profession of the 1940s

Before addressing the question directly, I would like to provide some relevant historical information. Carl Rogers (1902-1987) received his PhD in psychology from Columbia University in 1931 and spent his early professional years working in child guidance clinics. Originally, clinical psychologists had been associated primarily with intelligence and personality testing, but by the time Rogers came along in the late 1920s and 1930s some had begun to do "counseling" or "guidance." However, the "more serious" work of psychotherapy was still the domain of psychiatrists. Psychiatrists considered themselves the only ones capable of diagnosing and treating mental pathology because (a) they were physicians and (b) they had been trained in the complex and somewhat mysterious techniques of psychoanalysis. Psychiatrists were at the top of the professional hierarchy and psychologists, social workers, and psychiatric nurses were little more than "handmaidens" to psychiatrists. In short, psychiatrists held the power in the "mental health" field.

They also held the power in psychotherapy. Psychiatrists were the "experts" who "diagnosed" and "administered treatments" to "patients." In keeping with the medical model, the patient's job was to provide information and follow the doctor's orders. The doctor's job was to analyze the patient's material and make interpretations so that, in time, patients might gain insight into their own unconscious dynamics. Thus, as physician and trained analyst, the psychiatrist was "in charge" of the therapeutic relationship.

This was the historical stage onto which Carl Rogers walked in the early 1940s with his "non-directive" approach, as his theory was then called. Based on his research and clinical experience, Rogers had come to the conclusion that most clients are capable of arriving at their own insights and solving their own problems. He believed therapy was more successful when the counselor did not analyze, interpret, direct, control, or give advice but, instead, focused on the client's process and accepted, recognized, and helped clarify the client's feelings (see Bozarth et al., 2001; Cain, 2001a; Rogers, 1942). In short, Rogers rejected the therapist-centered model of therapy and articulated a new client-centered approach.

Rogers's views created an immediate uproar in the professional community, especially among psychiatrists. The idea that patients could solve their own problems without a psychotherapist to direct the therapy and to analyze and interpret the client's material was considered both naïve and dangerous. Even as late as 1951, at the prestigious Menninger Clinic, Rogers was told that his brand of therapy would create psychopaths (Rogers, 1977).

Rogers was puzzled by the negative reactions and wondered why his ideas were so upsetting. He assumed it was because the ideas were new and had come from a psychologist, not a psychiatrist. However, in the later years of his life, Rogers came across a concept that illumined these early experiences. In fact, the concept had such a profound impact on Rogers that it caused him to reassess all of his professional work. The concept was "the politics of interpersonal relationships." Rogers (1977) described how he was first exposed to this concept:

> Three years ago I was asked about the politics of the client-centered approach to psychotherapy. I replied that there was no politics in client-centered therapy, an answer which was greeted with a loud guffaw. When I asked my questioner to explain, he replied, "I spent three years of graduate school learning to be an expert in clinical psychology. I learned to make accurate diagnostic judgments. I learned the various techniques of altering the subject's attitude and behavior. I learned subtle modes of manipulation, under the labels of interpretation and guidance. Then I began to read your material, which upset everything I had learned. You were saying that the power rests not in my mind but in his organism. You completely reversed the relationship of power and control which had been built up in me over three years. And then you say there is no politics in the client-centered approach!" (p. 3)

At the time of this exchange, Rogers was unfamiliar with the word "politics" as a term to describe interpersonal relationships. Later, Rogers (1977) wrote:

The use of the word "politics" in such contexts as "the politics of the family," "the politics of therapy," "sexual politics," "the politics of experience" is new. I have not found any dictionary definition that even suggests the way in which the word is currently utilized.... Politics, in present-day psychological and social usage, has to do with power and control: with the extent to which persons desire, attempt to obtain, possess, share, or surrender power and control over others and/or themselves. (p. 4)

This new concept gave Rogers a way to understand why his ideas had created such furor in the 1940s. Rogers (1977) said:

It has taken me years to recognize that the violent opposition to a client-centered therapy sprang not only from its newness, and the fact that it came from a psychologist rather than a psychiatrist, but primarily because it struck such an outrageous blow to the therapist's *power*. It was in its *politics* that it was most threatening. (pp. 16-17)

A few pages earlier, Rogers (1977) had said:

I see now that I had dealt a double-edged political blow. I had said that most counselors saw themselves as competent to control the lives of their clients. And I had advanced the view that it was preferable simply to free the client to become an independent, self-directing person. I was making it clear that if they agreed with me, it would mean the complete disruption and reversal of their personal control in their counseling relationships. (pp. 6 -7)

Rogers's client-centered views turned the "politics" of psychotherapy upside down. Rogers had said that the *client*--not the therapist--was the expert on the client's problems. The *client*--not the therapist--had the ability to solve those problems. The *client*--not the therapist--held the power. Without fully realizing it at the time, Rogers had asked psychiatrists to give up their role as the "all-knowing doctor" and to focus, instead, on creating a therapeutic relationship characterized by empathy and acceptance that would free clients to grow and thus become capable of solving their own problems. In a sense, Rogers had asked psychiatrists to become "servants" to the client's process.[1] Clearly, in terms of the "politics of power," Rogers had hit psychiatrists where it hurt.

Carl Rogers and Contemporary Clinical Psychology

But what does this history have to do with the question of why Rogers is ignored by contemporary clinical psychology? I would suggest that, in large measure, Rogers is ignored today for the same reasons he was attacked by psychiatrists in the 1940s: His client-centered views represent a threat to contemporary clinical psychology just as they represented a threat to the psychiatric community in the 1940s. To adapt a campaign slogan, "It's the politics, Stupid."

Contemporary clinical psychology is committed to the medical model--the same model that dominated psychiatry in the 1940s. Most clinical psychologists view themselves as "doctors" who "diagnose" "mental disorders" and "administer treatments" to "patients." Thus, Rogers's view that psychotherapy is not a set of medical-like procedures but, rather, an interpersonal process that frees clients to grow and actualize their potentials is a threat to contemporary clinical psychology just as it was a threat to the psychiatric community 70 years ago. If clinical psychologists adopted Rogers's views, they would have to give up their role as "doctors" and the power this gives them over clients, along with their belief that their medical-like techniques are responsible for therapeutic effectiveness. Further, they would have to focus their therapeutic efforts on creating an empathic, accepting, and open relationship in which their clients could grow, discover their own insights, and find their own directions. For those who view themselves as "doctors" who "administer treatments," this is not easy to do. Even for those who are not invested in power and who are, in fact, drawn to Rogers's ideas, it is difficult to embrace and practice client-centered values. Our profession is so dominated by the medical model that in many clinical settings one's professional competence is judged by one's ability to speak medical jargon and to describe what one does in

---

[1] It is worth mentioning that, etymologically, the word "therapist" means "attendant" or "servant."

medical model terms. Also, adherents of the medical model tend to receive the professional and economic rewards (e.g., better jobs, promotions, salaries) that come to those who collaborate with the system. Thus, the politics of clinical psychology, including its medical model ideology and system of professional and economic rewards, makes it difficult for clinical psychologists to embrace Rogers's views even if they are inclined to do so. (For a more detailed critique of the medical model, see chapter four or Elkins, 2007).

And what about clinical training? Why do so many programs marginalize or ignore Rogers and his ideas? Again, I would suggest that, in large measure, it's the "politics." Most training programs in clinical psychology, like the rest of the profession, are immersed in the medical model. The academic courses and supervised training are designed to produce "doctors" who can "diagnose" "mental disorders" and "administer treatments" to "patients." Rogers's views simply do not fit in such programs. In fact, if his views were taken seriously, they would undermine the ideology and goals of these programs, not to mention how much they would upset professors who teach courses based on medical model assumptions. Also, imagine what would happen if a significant number of students were drawn to Rogers and his ideas. Suppose they said, "This is what we always thought psychotherapy should be." Clearly, this could create a serious morale problem, leading students to challenge their professors and to question the validity of their training experiences. Thus, in terms of the politics of power, it is in the best interest of most training programs in clinical psychology to ignore Rogers as much as possible.

Insights from the field of critical psychology are relevant here. Critical psychology, which began in Germany in 1970, is now a substantial movement (see Fox & Prilleltensky, 1997; Prilleltensky & Nelson, 2002; Slife, Reber, & Richardson, 2005). Critical psychologists are committed to social justice and examine, among other things, how psychology may collude, wittingly or unwittingly, with social and political forces that are harmful to human beings. For example, critical psychologists have raised concerns about clinical psychology's tendency to focus on individual pathology while ignoring the larger social forces that produce that pathology. Another issue they address--more directly related to this chapter--is how and why psychology sanctions some points of view but ignores or resists others. The term "gate-keepers" has been used to refer to those who exercise power in determining which ideas are "allowed in" and which are not. For example, influential psychology organizations such as the APA and editors of major psychology journals exercise considerable power in determining which ideas receive attention and which do not. Perhaps the most powerful gate-keepers, however, are training programs in clinical psychology. Because everyone who wishes to become a clinical psychologist must pass through their gates, training programs have enormous power to shape students' views of the profession and to indoctrinate them into whatever happens to be the dominant ideology of the profession. Because training programs want to retain their APA accreditation, be viewed positively by the professional community, and ensure that their students are able to function effectively in the "real world" of clinical psychology, they are motivated to provide conventional training so their students can secure conventional internships which will prepare them for conventional jobs in conventional settings. Thus, training programs have political and economic reasons to reflect the dominant ideology of the profession and to marginalize ideas that are not congruent with that ideology. As an example of how outside forces can affect clinical training, consider how quickly some programs reinvented themselves in the 1980s and 1990s to reflect managed care's emphasis on short-term therapies and "empirically supported treatments." The danger in allowing marketplace and other external forces to shape clinical training is that science and good critical thinking may be trumped by political and economic considerations. Indeed, scientific findings have now raised serious questions about the overly zealous claims made by adherents of short-term therapies and so-called "empirically supported treatments" (see Elkins, 2007, 2008; Hubble, Duncan, & Miller, 1999; Miller, 1994, 1996a, 1996b, 1996c; Seligman, 1995; Wampold, 2001).

I am not suggesting that those in charge of clinical training programs lie awake at night trying to think of ways to marginalize Carl Rogers. Instead, I am suggesting that training programs are caught in a web of political and economic forces that influence which ideas are considered acceptable and which are resisted. Thus, training programs can become centers of orthodoxy, dedicated to reflecting the status quo, instead of centers of creative and critical thinking that welcome alternative and innovative ideas. This political perspective makes it easier to understand why Rogers, one of the most important clinicians in history, is ignored. He is ignored because his ideas are inconsistent with, and represent a serious threat to, the medical model ideology that dominates contemporary clinical training and practice.

Rogers's Contributions and Their Political Implications

After his controversial debut in the 1940s, Rogers went on to become a leading figure in American psychology. Research on client-centered therapy and the studies it inspired literally dominated psychotherapy research for more than 20 years–from the early 1940s through the early 1960s (Bozarth et al., 2001). Eventually, hundreds of students, psychologists, counselors, social workers, family therapists, group therapists, and even a few psychiatrists embraced client-centered values. They were drawn to Rogers's view that clients have an innate ability to actualize their potentials and that certain therapeutic conditions release this actualizing tendency. While it is not the purpose of this chapter to discuss all of Rogers's contributions, it does seem important to highlight those that have political implications and are thus in line with the focus of this chapter. Three overlapping contributions and their political implications are discussed below.

Contextual Factors as the Effective Ingredients in Psychotherapy

During his tenure at the University of Chicago in the late 1940s and 1950s, Rogers came to believe that the "conditions" he had discovered in client-centered therapy (i.e., empathy, unconditional positive regard, and congruence) were the healing factors in all therapeutic systems (Rogers, 1957, 1959). Thus, the research moved beyond an exclusive focus on client-centered therapy and turned to the study of these conditions in other therapeutic approaches. Although we now know that "contextual factors" include more than Rogers's three conditions, contemporary research on contextual factors (e.g., Wampold, 2001) makes it clear that Rogers was on the right track to reject the medical model with its emphasis on techniques and to focus, instead, on other factors in the therapeutic situation as the effective ingredients in psychotherapy. This contribution of Rogers has political implications because, like the recent research on contextual factors, it represents a frontal attack on the medical model and its focus on techniques as the determinants of therapeutic outcome.

Rogers's Theory of Interpersonal Relationships

During the 1950s Rogers and his associates broadened the focus of their research beyond psychotherapy to include other interpersonal relationships such as parent-child, teacher-student, and employer-employee (see Gordon, 1970; Montuori & Purser, 2001; Thomas, 2001). As research findings came in, it became increasingly clear that Rogers had discovered a simple formula with revolutionary potential to transform human relationships: *If those in positions of authority are willing to relinquish their power over others and create an interpersonal milieu characterized by empathy, respect, and congruence, amazing things are likely to happen. When individuals realize that they are free to exercise their own power and develop their own potentials, they tend to come alive and to grow in unpredictable but deeply meaningful ways.* This new theory had powerful political implications because it challenged authoritarian and paternalistic models of human relationships and supported the power of children, students, employees, women, ethnic minorities, and others whom society has often consigned to subordinate positions in terms of power.

A New Theory of Power

Early on, Rogers's research and clinical experience caused him to reject therapist-centered approaches that focused on guiding, advising, suggesting, and persuading clients. His subsequent research confirmed that clients tend to move in positive, therapeutic directions when therapists relinquish their control and support the power of the client. From a historical perspective, Rogers was challenging the authoritarian and paternalistic view of the therapeutic relationship that had originated with Freud in the Victorian Age. This is the same view of human relationships that once led our society to believe that husbands should have power over wives, that whites should dominate blacks, that missionaries should "Christianize" traditional cultures, and that the U.S. government should "civilize" Native Americans. It does not matter that there may have been some good husbands, whites, missionaries, and government agents. It is also irrelevant that some of the oppressed may have liked, loved, befriended, or collaborated with their oppressors. *What made these systems inherently flawed and irredeemably immoral was their "politics"–the authoritarian and paternalistic assumption that certain groups know what is best for others and therefore have a right to exercise power over them.* Such systems not only violate basic human rights but they also limit or destroy the unique potentials of those who are oppressed. Authoritarian and paternalistic systems–including therapy administered by experts who think they know what is best for others-- are far more dangerous than we have been led to believe.

Psychotherapy is highly political in the sense that it wields enormous power in clients' lives. In therapy, clients make decisions that change their lives forever; they set sail on existential journeys of no return. Thus, how we as therapists deal with the power inherent in psychotherapy is vitally important. As Rogers recognized, there are two basic choices: We can assume the role of "expert" and tell clients how to solve their problems and live their lives or we can adopt an emancipatory approach that supports clients' power and frees them to make their own decisions, solve their own problems, find their own directions, and become more fully who they are. As Rogers (1942) put it:

> Therapy is not a matter of doing something to the individual or of inducing him to do something about himself. It is instead a matter of freeing him for normal growth and development, of removing obstacles so that he can again move forward. (pp. 28-29)

Referring to Gertrude Stein's famous statement about the city of Paris, "It is not what Paris gives you but what she does not take away," Rogers (1977) said, "This can be paraphrased to become a definition of the person-centered approach.... It is not that this approach gives power to the person; it never takes it away" (p. xii).

This contribution has political implications because it challenges therapists to abandon paternalistic approaches that disempower and to embrace emancipatory approaches that set clients free. It is difficult to imagine how one can truly respect the power of clients while relating to them as a "doctor" who "diagnoses" their "pathology" and "administers treatments" to "cure" their "mental disorders." We have become so accustomed to such medical model language that we often fail to see just how patronizing and disempowering it is. In contrast, Rogers's approach to therapy, along with other emancipatory approaches, supports the client's power and adamantly refuses to take it away. (For an excellent discussion of emancipatory therapy, see O'Hara, 2001).

Concluding Thoughts: Where We Are Today

Despite Rogers's research which showed that interpersonal factors--not techniques--were the effective ingredients in psycho-therapy, clinical psychology made a radical turn in the 1970s toward investigations of "specificity," i.e., specific treatments for specific disorders (see Bergin, 1997; Bozarth, et al., 2001). Why this change occurred is not clear, but it certainly was not based on previous research findings. Most likely, it represented a resurgence of the medical model in the vacuum created when Rogers and his associates completed their last major research project in the 1960s (see Gendlin, Kieseler, Rogers, & Truax, 1967). Also, many researchers and clinicians, perhaps because of their "hard science" training, have difficulty believing that something as "soft" as relational factors can be responsible for therapeutic effectiveness, even though the research has confirmed this again and again. Whatever the reasons, the research tradition that Rogers had originated and that had dominated clinical research for more than two decades went into eclipse in the United States in the 1970s, and for the next 25 years (from the mid-1970s to the late 1990s) specificity research took center stage, bolstered in the 1980s and 1990s by the rise of managed care with its medical model assumptions about psychotherapy and its insistence that clinical psychologists demonstrate the scientific validity of their techniques (see Bozarth et al., 2001, Elkins, 2007).

Today, however, something new is happening. After 25 years of specificity research that involved thousands of efficacy studies and millions of research dollars, clinical researchers have failed to demonstrate that any particular technique is any more effective than any other technique (Ahn & Wampold, 2001; Elkins, 2007; Messer & Wampold, 2000; Wampold, 1997, 2001, 2005). Equally dramatic, recent analyses and meta-analyses of thousands of research studies conducted over several decades have made it clear that contextual factors--not techniques--are the primary determinants of therapeutic outcome (see Asay & Lambert, 1999; Elkins, 2008; Hubble et al., 1999; Wampold et al., 1997; Wampold, 2001, 2005, 2007). The term "contextual factors" refers to such elements as the alliance, the relationship, the personal qualities and interpersonal skills of the therapist, client agency, patient expectations, extra-therapeutic factors, and so on. These findings, which are a devastating blow to the medical model with its focus on techniques, are slowly forcing clinical psychology to revisit the idea that certain factors common to all therapeutic systems are the effective ingredients in psychotherapy. This is a powerful vindication of Rogers's work and shows that he was correct to reject the medical model with its emphasis on techniques and to focus on personal and interpersonal factors as major determinants of therapeutic outcome. Thus, the eclipse that placed Rogers and his research findings in semi-darkness for more than 25 years is now over and it is time for clinical psychology to revisit Rogers in the context of contemporary research on contextual factors. The only thing that could prevent us from doing this is our irrational dedication to the medical model and the recalcitrant politics of our profession.

"Whatever happened to Carl Rogers?" Perhaps the best answer is this: He was about 50 years ahead of his time and has been waiting for us to catch up.

Because we now know that longer-term therapy is, on the whole, more effective than short-term approaches, we need to raise questions about the ethical implications of training programs, internship sites, and psychology clinics collaborating with a system that harms thousands of clients by rationing treatment and denying them the longer-term therapy they need.

.

Chapter Two

Short-Term, Linear Approaches to Psychotherapy
What We Now Know

Chapter Overview: The chapter describes the inherent weaknesses of short-term, linear approaches, summarizes research showing they are less effective than longer-term, traditional psychotherapy, and examines the political and economic forces that created them and keep them in place. The author encourages those who are drawn to short-term, linear approaches to embed them in a more complex theoretical framework such as that which humanistic-existential (HE) psychology provides.

In this day of managed care and short-term therapies, many clinical settings have adopted a linear approach to psychotherapy. By "linear" I mean clear-cut, sequential, and streamlined. After one or two sessions, the clinician is required to write a treatment plan specifying the problems to be addressed, the techniques that will be used to address each problem, and the criteria to determine when therapy is complete. The therapy itself, which is time-limited and focused on clinical efficiency, consists of techniques, homework assignments, progress reports from the client, and adjustments in the techniques and assignments as needed to alleviate the problems specified in the treatment plan. This short-term, linear approach to psychotherapy is appealing. It is immediately understandable by clients and it gives therapists a clear sense of where they are, where they're going, how to get there, and what to do in each session. The approach appeals to managed care companies looking for ways to contain costs, to grant-funded clinics that must describe in clear language what they do, to boards that oversee mental health institutions, and to politicians who vote on bills related to mental health. On top of all this, proponents have claimed that research shows short-term, linear approaches are just as effective as traditional therapy for most clients (Bloom, 1992; Budman & Gurman, 1983, 1988; Koss & Butcher, 1986; Koss & Shiang, 1994; Luborksy, Singer, & Luborsky, 1975; Steenbarger, 1994). Thus, short-term, linear approaches seem to cover all the bases. *Nevertheless, I will show in this chapter that short-term, linear approaches have inherent limitations, that the research shows they are not as effective as longer-term therapy, that they have proliferated in recent years not because they are more effective but because of managed care's focus on treatment rationing, and that they are based on a fundamental misunderstanding of the nature of emotional suffering and therapeutic healing.*

Limitations of Short-Term, Linear Approaches

Short-term, linear approaches have several inherent limitations. First, they are based on a "problem solving" model that is more associated with American corporate thinking than with client suffering and therapeutic healing. Typically, the model includes the following sequence: (a) identify the problem, (b) consider various interventions to solve the problem, (c) choose the best interventions, (d) apply the interventions, (e) assess progress periodically, and (f) modify the interventions as needed. This clear-cut, linear approach appeals to executives, administrators, and others in positions of authority and has proven itself effective as an approach to solving problems in corporate and other settings. It is no accident that the trend toward streamlined, linear approaches in clinical work coincided with the rise of managed care and its corporate mentality (Ackley, 1997; Miller, 1996c). Not only did managed care bring about a proliferation of linear approaches in psychotherapy, but it also brought about the reorganization of training programs and treatment centers to coincide with these approaches. Doctoral students and psychologists have learned that to get an internship or a job in many mental health settings requires one to hide psychodynamic or humanistic leanings and to declare one's undying commitment to short-term, linear approaches!

While it is tempting to jump on the short-term, linear bandwagon, I would suggest that psychologists and students look before they leap. There is growing evidence that the bandwagon is having serious difficulties (Howard, Kopta, Krause, & Orlinsky, 1986; Howard, Lueger, Maling, & Martinovich, 1993; Luborsky, Chandler, Auerback, Cohen, & Bachrach, 1971; Orlinsky & Howard, 1986; Miller, 1994, 1996a, 1996b, 1996c; Seligman, 1995; Westen & Morrison, 2001). The main problem seems to be this: Emotional suffering and therapeutic healing cannot be forced into a short-term, linear format. Corporate America may be good at streamlined problem-solving and efficient organization, but it knows little or nothing about emotional suffering and the complexities of therapeutic healing. Instead of jumping on the bandwagon and supporting the short-term, linear trend, psychologists should persistently voice concerns about managed care and its economically-motivated emphasis on treatment rationing and short-term therapies. Because we now know that longer-term therapy is, on the whole, more effective than short-term approaches, we need to raise questions about the ethical implications of training programs, internship sites, and psychology clinics collaborating with a system that harms thousands of clients by rationing treatment and denying them the longer-term therapy they need. We must not sell out on traditional psychotherapy and clients' needs for a mess of corporate pottage!

Second, streamlined treatment plans formulated after one or two sessions make little sense from a sophisticated, clinical perspective. Such plans are based on the assumption that a therapist has the ability--in one or two sessions--to figure out what the client's problems are and how to solve them. I would suggest that no clinician, regardless how perceptive, has this ability. The real problems of a client may not surface until many weeks into the therapy. It is not so much that clients intentionally hide the truth from the therapist (although this also happens) but rather that clients themselves often don't know what the real problem is. This is not a paternalistic statement about the client's lack of insight but a realistic description of the nature of emotional suffering. A female client may state that she has come to therapy because she is experiencing stress due to her demanding job when in reality the problem is that she is in a marriage where she receives little understanding or support. The difficulties in the marriage, which are the real problem, may not come to the surface in a therapy that is dominated by a treatment plan that identifies "stress due to her demanding job" as the problem and focuses on techniques and homework assignments designed to alleviate that stress.

If clinicians cannot divine a client's problems in one or two initial sessions, then any treatment plan based on information gained in those sessions is clinically naïve at best and dangerous at worst. Clinicians who, because of institutional demands or their own clinical naiveté, assume that the presenting problem is always the real problem may spend the ensuing therapy sessions dealing with pseudo-problems and never get to the client's real problems. Of course, short-term, linear therapists would argue that they are not bound to the original treatment plan and can change directions if other problems surface in the course of treatment. The trouble, however, is that in a short-term, technique-dominated therapy, where the focus is on the problem at hand, there may be little time or opportunity for the client to do the kind of self-exploration required to unearth the deeper problems. Thus, while linear treatment plans formulated after one or two sessions may look good on paper, they are unsophisticated from a clinical perspective because they fail to take into account the complex nature of human personality, emotional suffering, and therapeutic healing.

As Freud discovered and thousands of clinicians have confirmed in their own practices, good psychotherapy is *precisely* about helping clients discover their real problems. The dynamic insights, emotional release, and cognitive restructuring that occur when a client finally faces the deeper truths of his or her life are at the very heart of the healing process. In the Greek language there are various words for "truth." The word *aletheia* (pronounced ah-lay-thay-ah) refers to the kind of truth that is revealed when one goes below surface appearances to a deeper level. Art provides excellent illustrations of this kind of truth. For example, Van Gogh's painting "The Potato Eaters" is, at the surface level, simply a depiction of a few rough-looking people sitting around a table and eating potatoes. At a deeper level, however, the painting reveals the universal pain, hunger, and ennui of those who live in abject poverty. This deeper truth is the truth known as *aletheia*. Martin Heidegger (1977), using his philosophical language of beings and Being, talked about *aletheia* as "unconcealedness." Referring to another painting by Van Gogh that depicts a pair of peasant shoes, Heidegger wrote:

> Van Gogh's painting is the disclosure of what the equipment, the pair of peasant shoes, *is* in truth. This being emerges into the unconcealedness of its Being. The Greeks called the unconcealedness of beings *aletheia*. We say "truth" and think little enough in using this word. If there occurs in the work a disclosure of a particular being, disclosing what and how it is, then there is here an occurring, a happening of truth at work. (p. 164)

Aletheia also describes a certain kind of human relationship. Let's say, for example, that you know a person at work but your relationship is only a surface relationship. Then one day, perhaps while working on a project together, the two of you begin to talk. At first, you discuss surface topics but then the conversation moves to a deeper level. To use Heidegger's word, "unconcealedness" occurs as you open yourselves to each other. The relationship moves to a deeper, "truer" level. This is the realm of *aletheia,* a deeper kind of relationship and a deeper kind of truth.

In psychotherapy *aletheia* is the kind of truth that clients often discover when they go beneath the presenting problem to explore the deeper truths of their lives. It is not that the presenting problem is necessarily "false" but rather that it's a surface problem. Indeed, it may even serve as a cover for the *real* problems that lie at a deeper, less accessible level. Psychotherapy is about *aletheia*, the discovery of the deeper truths that underlie clients' suffering (as well as the strengths and potentials they may not know they possess). Treatment plans based on surface truths solve surface problems and may never reach the level of *aletheia*.

Carl Rogers understood this. Although he did not use the term *aletheia*, he described how clients in psychotherapy gradually move from surface concerns to deeper levels. In *On Becoming a Person*, Rogers discussed how clients remove their "false faces" and "masks" as they move toward the core self. Rogers (1961) said:

This exploration becomes even more disturbing whenever they (clients) find themselves involved in removing the false faces which they had not known were false faces. They begin to engage in the frightening task of exploring the turbulent and sometimes violent feelings within themselves. To remove a mask which you had thought was part of your real self can be a deeply disturbing experience, yet when there is freedom to think and feel and be, the individual moves toward such a goal. (p. 110)

Rogers then presented a statement from one of his clients who had experienced this movement from the surface to the depths. The client's metaphor-filled description of her own process puts flesh and bones on the abstract notion of *aletheia*. The client said:

As I look at it now, I was peeling off layer after layer of defenses. I'd build them up, try them, and then discard them when you remained the same. I didn't know what was at the bottom and I was very much afraid to find out, but I had to keep on trying. At first I felt there was nothing within me--just a great emptiness where I needed and wanted a solid core. Then I began to feel that I was facing a solid brick wall, too high to get over and too thick to go through. One day the wall became translucent, rather than solid. After this, the wall seemed to disappear but beyond it I discovered a dam holding back violent, churning waters. I felt as if I were holding back the force of these waters and if I opened even a tiny hole I and all about me would be destroyed in the ensuing torrent of feelings represented by the water. Finally, I could stand the strain no longer and I let go. All I did, actually, was to succumb to complete and utter self pity, then hate, then love. After this experience, I felt as if I had leaped a brink and was safely on the other side, though still tottering a bit on the edge. I don't know what I was searching for or where I was going, but I felt then as I have always felt whenever I really lived, that I was moving forward. (p. 110)

Clearly, there is a profound difference between this kind of "*aletheia*-oriented" therapy in which the client moves from surface concerns to a deeper, more authentic level and the short-term, technique-focused treatments that now dominate our profession.

Third, despite claims to the contrary, research indicates that short-term, linear treatments may have limited effectiveness. Cognitive-Behavioral Therapy (CBT) is the sine qua non of short-term, linear approaches to psychotherapy so it is important to address CBT specifically. Historically, humanistic-existential (HE) psychologists criticized behavioral approaches as being based on a mechanistic image of the human being and on an "expert-doing-something-to-a-client" model of therapy. While these criticisms still have merit, they were more cogent in the 1950s and 1960s when applied to Watsonian behaviorism and Skinnerian operant conditioning. The cognitive focus of today's CBT is a far cry from Watsonian behaviorism, which viewed the mind as nothing but an epiphenomenon, and today's cognitive-behavioral therapists are far more collaborative in their therapeutic style than were the Skinnerian "behavior modification" experts of the past. Thus, I see nothing inherently contradictory about HE psychologists using a carefully considered cognitive and behavioral rationale, along with CBT procedures, as *one part* of an overall therapeutic approach. However, when CBT is elevated to the status of an exclusive and "total approach" to psychotherapy, I have several concerns. First, as discussed above, short-term, linear approaches including CBT may focus on surface or pseudo-problems and never get to the deeper issues of the client.

Second, CBT tends to focus on techniques and not give sufficient attention to the nature and quality of the therapeutic relationship and its power to heal. While some practitioners of CBT now put more emphasis on empathy because of research showing that empathic cognitive-behavioral therapists are more effective (Wampold, 2001), the primary focus remains on the techniques and procedures of the treatment, not on the therapeutic relationship. This is problematic because it now appears that specific techniques, within themselves, have little to do with therapeutic effectiveness whereas the therapeutic relationship is a powerful determinant of therapeutic outcome. Wampold's (2001) careful analyses and meta-analyses of the research confirmed that while the therapeutic relationship has a strong effect on therapeutic outcome, specific techniques have little, if anything at all, to do with therapeutic effectiveness. These findings undermine CBT's focus on techniques as the instruments of client improvement and raise serious questions about our profession's efforts to identify "empirically-supported" techniques. In other words, if specific techniques have little or nothing to do with client improvement, then the search for empirically supported techniques is misguided. The profession would be better served if researchers focused their efforts on discovering and clarifying therapeutic factors clearly responsible for client improvement. Because of the abundant research showing the importance of the therapeutic relationship in client improvement, Division 29, Psychotherapy, of the American Psychological Association, established the "Task Force on Empirically-Supported Therapy Relationships" to identify and present this information. After presenting the empirical evidence showing that the therapeutic relationship is a major determinant of therapeutic effectiveness, the task force called for greater emphasis on "empirically-supported relationships" (ESRs) to counterbalance the current emphasis on "empirically-supported treatments" (ESTs). (See Norcross, 2002, for a comprehensive presentation of the task force's work and Chapter Four of this book or Elkins, 2007, for a detailed discussion of so-called "empirically supported treatments").

Third, CBT focuses primarily on the individual's thoughts and behaviors and pays inadequate attention to the existential, familial, societal, ethnic, cultural, and spiritual factors that may contribute to, or even be at the root of, the client's difficulties. One reason CBT neglects these factors, no doubt, is that they are "messy" (i.e., complex) and do not fit easily into a linear approach. In addition, cognitive-behavioral therapists are committed to using "empirically validated" techniques and, the truth is, no such techniques exist for these messy, complex influences. Because cognitive-behavioral therapists tend to focus on client phenomena that can be treated with specific techniques, they tend to overlook or marginalize client phenomena that do not fit these techniques. Being more "method-centered" than "client-centered," CBT is often a hammer in search of a nail, ignoring phenomena that are not "hammer friendly."

Fourth, although CBT trainees typically receive intense training in specific techniques and procedures, they receive relatively little training in the personal, interpersonal, and artistic skills needed to honor the inherent "messiness" (i.e., complexity) of psychotherapy and to work effectively with it.

Fifth, CBT is not as "empirically-validated" as we have been led to believe. After completing an elaborate meta-analysis of research studies published in major journals on short-term, "empirically-supported therapies" used in the treatment of depression, generalized anxiety disorder, and panic, Westen and Morrison (2001) raised serious questions about the effectiveness of these approaches. The findings of this meta-analysis are summarized below.

The Westen and Morrison Meta-Analysis

Westen and Morrison (2001) completed a meta-analysis of 34 research studies on short-term, "empirically supported therapies" that were published in high quality journals from 1990 to 1998. The 34 studies, which involved 2,414 clients, included 12 studies of depression, 17 studies of panic, and 5 studies of generalized anxiety disorder. The following is a summary of their findings:

First, Westen and Morrison found that researchers often used such stringent exclusion criteria in selecting their subjects that the samples may bear little resemblance to the actual client population seen by therapists. Specifically, the authors found that prospective subjects with more than one diagnosis were often excluded from studies even though research shows that the majority of clients who seek psychotherapy have multiple problems and more than one diagnosis (Seligman, 1995). This raises serious questions about the generalizability of the findings to the actual clinical population seen by therapists.

Second, even with these "clean" samples, Westen and Morrison found that the improvement rates were generally low with regard to depression (54%) and generalized anxiety disorder (52%) for those who completed treatment. This finding is important because we have been told that CBT is highly effective in the treatment of these disorders, particularly depression.

Third, the improvement rate for panic was a more respectable 63% for those who completed treatment, suggesting that CBT is effective in treating panic.

Fourth, the authors found that follow-up studies (at 12 months, 24 months, etc.) were so seldom done by researchers that one could not draw any scientific conclusions about the long-term efficacy of the treatments for depression and generalized anxiety disorder. The meta-analysis did reveal empirical data to indicate CBT is effective in decreasing panic attacks, even over time.

Keep in mind that Westen and Morrison analyzed 34 studies involving more than 2,400 clients that were published in major journals over nearly a decade (1990-1998) that spanned the heyday of managed care and short-term, linear approaches. Yet, the only thing the authors could conclude from a scientific perspective was that CBT was effective in regard to the treatment of panic. Even this conclusion should be guarded, however, because of the problems with subject selection discussed above.

Westen and Morrison made two other points worth noting here: First, they distinguished between "states" and "disorders." To clarify, the authors gave an example of a client who is in a suicidal state. Emergency intervention might change the suicidal state, but one would not assume that the underlying problem or disorder had been solved simply because the client was no longer feeling suicidal. This distinction between states and disorders is helpful and raises important questions. For example, in the treatment of depression, do short-term, linear approaches help alleviate the depressive *state* but not necessarily the depressive *disorder* (i.e., the deeper problems causing the depression)? Also, do "checklist" instruments such as the Beck Depression Inventory (BDI) sometimes measure the client's depressive *state* but not necessarily the client's depressive *disorder* and, if so, how would one tell the difference? (For other concerns about the BDI, see Wampold, 2001). And finally, do we need longer-term and more complex therapeutic approaches to address the deeper problems associated with depression and other emotional problems? These are not rhetorical questions but they are questions that deserve answers because they raise serious concerns about short-term, linear approaches.

Second, Westen and Morrison noted that in the literature proponents of scientific techniques often criticize other therapeutic approaches as being "unscientific." The authors pointed out, however, that this thinking contains a logical error. One cannot say that a therapeutic approach is "unscientific" until it has been thoroughly tested. Thus, the authors suggest that it would be more appropriate to call an approach "untested" instead of "unscientific." If tested, some of the approaches that have been called unscientific may actually prove to be more effective than short-term, linear approaches such as

CBT. Indeed, as will be discussed below, there is now convincing evidence that longer-term therapy is more effective than short-term therapy (Miller, 1996c; Seligman, 1995).

While none of us wants to admit that our therapeutic approach is "unscientific" or even "untested," the truth is that all theoretical orientations, including CBT, have a long way to go before proponents can talk with scientific confidence about an "empirically-validated" approach in psychotherapy. Indeed, many humanistic-existential psychologists believe the quest for empirically-validated techniques is misguided and based on a fundamental misunderstanding of how therapy works and how science should be applied to the therapeutic arena (see Task Force for the Development of Practice Recommendations for the Provision of Humanistic Psychosocial Services, 2004; Wampold, 2001).

It is not my intention to be overly critical of CBT. I have the same concerns about psychodynamic and humanistic-existential therapists who revamp their therapies to fit the short-term, linear trend. Let's be clear that this trend did not occur because therapists across the land suddenly had a mass epiphany and realized that short-term, linear approaches are clinically more effective. *Instead, the trend toward short-term, linear approaches in psychotherapy has occurred because therapists and institutions are worried that in a managed care world they will not get their share of the economic pie unless they revamp everything and jump on the short-term, linear bandwagon* (Ackley, 1997; Miller, 1996c). In other words, the economic tail is wagging the clinical dog. And while it is understandable that clinicians, graduate psychology programs, internship settings, and mental health clinics want to stay in business, it is also true that jumping on the bandwagon and helping the tail wag the dog are probably not the best ways to deal with managed care and its intrusion into the therapeutic arena.

Other Studies That Raise Concerns About Short-Term, Linear Approaches

If the meta-analysis by Westen and Morrison (2001) was the only research raising concerns about short-term, linear approaches to psychotherapy, managed care and other proponents of short-term approaches might be able to ignore the study or explain it away.

However, other studies have come to similar conclusions about the limitations of short-term therapy and the claims for its effectiveness. Two of these studies are discussed below.

The Miller Study: A Critique of Time-Limited Therapy

Miller (1996c) revisited and carefully examined 16 research studies often cited to support the claim that time-limited therapies are as effective as traditional psychotherapy for the majority of clients. Miller pointed out that this claim has been made extensively in the literature by proponents of managed care and time-limited approaches. To illustrate, he quoted Bloom (1992), a proponent of short-term therapy, who went so far as to say that:

> ...without exception, empirical studies of short-term outpatient psychotherapy ...have found that planned short-term psychotherapies are essentially equally effective and are, in general, as effective as time-unlimited psychotherapy, virtually regardless of diagnosis **or** duration of treatment. Indeed, perhaps no other finding has been reported with greater regularity in the mental health literature than the equivalence of effect of time-limited and time-unlimited psychotherapy. (p. 9)

Miller then cited nine other reviews from 1975 to 1994 that had come to the same conclusion as did Bloom. This led Miller (1996c) to say:

> At this point, proponents of time limits have repeated their declarations of research support so many times that it appears to be established fact. But as I will show in the following review, on examination the research support for time limits vanishes, and the actual research evidence shows that time limits are harmful. The belief that research supports time limits has only survived because the evidence was never closely scrutinized. (p. 568)

Miller then reported the results of his examination of the studies often cited to support short-term approaches. The following is a summary of his findings:

First, Miller discovered that the claims for short-term therapy being as effective as traditional therapy were based on a small number of studies. Miller located 16 studies. Two others, which he was unable to locate, were unpublished papers presented at conferences in 1967 and 1978.

Second, Miller found that most of the reviews simply accepted and repeated the findings of two earlier reviews: Johnson and Gelso (1980) and Luborsky, Singer, and Luborsky (1975).

Third, when he examined the 16 studies used to support short-term claims, Miller discovered major problems with many of the studies. For example, 11 were incorrectly classified. Seven did not address the comparison of time-limited therapy (TLT) and clinically determined treatment (CDT) and should never have been cited as supporting time-limited therapy. One study had been published or reviewed as three independent studies and when Miller examined the original study, he found that the results, correctly interpreted, actually supported CDT as more effective than TLT. Miller found that the results of two studies were reported incorrectly and that, once again, the results actually supported the superiority of CDT over TLT. In short, Miller's examination of these studies deconstructed in a rather devastating way the often-repeated claim that short-term therapy is as effective as traditional therapy.

Fourth, Miller found that only five studies of the 16 had been properly classified and actually addressed the comparison of CDT and TLT. Incredibly, four out of the five studies, correctly interpreted, showed that CDT was more effective than TLT! Even the fifth study "leaned" in the direction of CDT but did not reach statistical significance. (Miller noted that it was a small study involving 29 clients and that the difference in the length of therapy for the two comparison groups was only four sessions).

Fifth, the only studies Miller found that supported the effectiveness of short-term therapy as being equal to or greater than traditional therapy was a 1969 study that used family treatment as the modality. The results showed TLT to be more effective than CDT on several measures. However, a replication study in 1973 found a difference on one measure: husband improvement.

Sixth, as for individual psychotherapy, Miller did not find even one study that supported the effectiveness of short-term therapy as being equal to or greater than traditional, "clinically determined" therapy.

Seventh, Miller discussed the so-called *Consumers Reports* study reported by Seligman (1995) in the *American Psychologist*. Miller noted that this study, along with the four mentioned above, showed that longer-term therapy was more effective than short-term therapy. Because this study is summarized below, I will not discuss it here.

Despite Miller's finding that short-term therapy is not as effective as longer-term therapy, he nevertheless supports the use of short-term approaches when they are clinically determined and clinically appropriate. Listing situations where brief therapy would be indicated, Miller (1996c) named "crisis intervention, a request for consultation and education, an evaluation, a response to clients with limited goals, the treatment of clients who are psychologically ready for a rapid change, and the treatment of conditions that respond quickly." (p. 567). Miller believes therapists should be trained in both short-term and long-term strategies so they can competently provide the kind of therapy required by the client's situation. As he put it:

> The therapist who is not trained in short-term techniques will not be able to offer these when they would be effective. Alternatively, the therapist who is not trained in long-term techniques will not be able to offer these when they are necessary. Both an increased diversity of training and an increased diversity of available professionals can lead to providing treatment closer to the optimal length. (p. 575)

Miller's work is an important contribution. He dismantled, study-by-study, the purported evidence for the claim that short-term therapy is as effective as traditional therapy. Going further, he demonstrated that the research actually showed just the opposite to be true: longer-term, clinically-determined therapy is more effective than time-limited therapy. The following statement by Miller (1996c) sums up his findings in this regard:

> Correctly interpreted, the research shows that time-limited treatment is inferior to psychotherapy in which the treatment time is clinically determined....The evidence indicates that

time limits merely curtail treatment before optimal benefits are achieved, and, for some clients, before psychologically necessary gains are accomplished. (p. 567)

Seligman's Consumers Reports *Study: Summary of Findings*

Another study that demonstrated the superiority of longer-term therapy is the so-called *Consumers Reports* study. The study was based on responses to a survey by 2,900 readers of *Consumers Reports* who had seen a mental health professional in the past three years for stress or other emotional problems. The results were published in *Consumers Reports* (1995) and Seligman (1995), who served as a consultant for the study, published an article about the research and its findings in the *American Psychologist*. Seligman's article described the survey questionnaire, the methods of the study, and the statistical analyses performed. He pointed out the advantages of the study, which focused on therapy as it is actually practiced and experienced in the field, over traditional efficacy studies that compare a particular treatment to a comparison group under controlled conditions. Seligman (1995), who had earlier supported efficacy studies as the ideal, said:

> I no longer believe that efficacy studies are the only, or even the best, way of finding out what treatments actually work in the field. I have come to believe that the "effectiveness" study of how patients fare under the actual conditions of treatment in the field can yield useful and credible "empirical validation" of psychotherapy and medication. This is the method that *Consumers Reports* pioneered. (p. 966)

In addition to discussing its advantages, Seligman also discussed the limitations and potential limitations of the study. While acknowledging that the study was not without flaws, he convincingly demonstrated that it was a sound study, worthy of our attention. As Seligman (1995) put it:

> The *Consumer Reports* study, then, is to be taken seriously--not only for its results and its credible source, but for its method. It is large-scale; it samples treatment as it is actually delivered in the field; it samples without obvious bias those

who seek out treatment; it measures multiple outcomes including specific improvement and more global gains such as growth, insight, productivity, mood, enjoyment of life, and interpersonal relations; it is statistically stringent and finds clinically meaningful results. (p. 974)

The following is a summary of the major findings: First, the study showed that psychotherapy worked. Of the 786 respondents who reported feeling *fairly poor* at the outset of therapy, 92% said they felt *very good*, *good*, or at least *so-so* by the time of the survey. Even more dramatic, of the 486 respondents who reported feeling *very poor* at the start of therapy, 87% reported that they felt *very good*, *good*, or at least *so-so* by the time of the survey, with 54% reporting that treatment *made things a lot better* and another third saying that it *made things somewhat better*. Thus, the findings indicate that the majority of respondents who were treated by a mental health professional showed improvement, with many showing very significant improvement. These findings support numerous other analyses and meta-analyses of the research that show conclusively that psychotherapy is effective (See Wampold, 2001, for information on this body of research).

Second, the study clearly showed that longer-term therapy resulted in more improvement than short-term therapy. Seligman (1995) said, "This result was very robust and held up over all statistical models" (p. 968). In Seligman's article, a bar graph was used to illustrate the relationship of improvement and duration of treatment. The duration axis was divided into increments of less than 1 month, 1-2 months, 3-6 months, 7-11 months, 1-2 years, and more than 2 years. At every increment of increased duration the graph showed increased improvement, suggesting that client improvement does not quickly "top out" in psychotherapy and that there are significant benefits to be gained by clients in longer-term therapy.

Third, the findings indicated that psychotherapy by itself was just as effective as psychotherapy plus medication (e.g., Prozac or Xanax) for any disorder. This finding is important in light of concerns about the overuse of psychiatric drugs and the current efforts to secure prescription privileges for psychologists. Based on this study, one might wonder why some psychologists are so adamant about securing prescription privileges when the clinical interventions this privilege would make possible would apparently add little, if anything, to psychotherapy. It might be better if psychologists focused their time and energy on improving their psychotherapeutic skills and leaving prescription privileges to psychiatrists and other adherents of the medical model. In cases such as schizophrenia, bipolar disorder, and severe depression, where medication might be indicated, psychologists can refer the client to a psychiatrist or physician, as we have done for decades. Of course, if the drive for prescription privileges is motivated primarily by economic and "turf" considerations, this would explain why this finding has had no detectable effect on the push for prescription privileges.

Fourth, the study found no significant difference in the therapeutic effectiveness of psychiatrists, psychologists, and social workers. All were equally able to help clients improve. Marriage counselors and physicians were also helpful, but their effectiveness was less than that of psychiatrists, psychologists, and social workers.

Fifth, the study found that no particular kind of therapy did any better than any other kind of therapy. This finding supports the research of Wampold (2001) who concluded, based on analyses and meta-analyses of studies of therapeutic effectiveness, that the kind of therapy and the specific ingredients of therapeutic systems have little, if anything, to do with therapeutic effectiveness. Instead, Wampold found that therapeutic effectiveness is the result of certain factors that are common to all therapeutic systems. For example, the therapeutic alliance, which is common to all therapeutic systems, is a powerful determinant of therapeutic effectiveness, whereas specific ingredients, i.e., the techniques and procedures of a particular modality, have little, if any, effect on therapeutic outcome. The *Consumers Reports* study supports this conclusion.

Overall, the *Consumers Reports* study, which was the largest survey ever conducted on the effectiveness of psychotherapy, made important contributions to our understanding of psychotherapy as it is practiced and experienced in the field. In specific regard to this article, the study showed clearly that longer-term therapy is more effective than short-term therapy.

Conclusion

In light of the information and research presented in this chapter, I would encourage psychology students, beginning therapists, and others who are drawn to short-term, linear approaches to consider embedding these in a broader, more complex therapeutic framework such as that which humanistic-existential psychology provides. Historically, HE psychology welcomed diverse therapeutic approaches and there is no reason that it cannot integrate CBT and other short-term approaches into its framework. In *The Psychology of Existence: An Integrative, Clinical Perspective*, Rollo May and Kirk Schneider (1995; see also Schneider, 2007) discussed the importance of an integrative approach. This does not mean that HE psychology should "swallow whole" any therapeutic approach that comes along, but it does mean that we should always be open to a careful, thoughtful integration of any perspective that does not, within itself, undermine humanistic principles and that can make useful contributions to the therapeutic endeavor. HE psychology can offer those who are drawn to short-term, linear approaches some important antidotes to the limitations of short-term, linear approaches as discussed in this chapter. Specifically, HE psychology can help students, beginning therapists, and others to (a) free themselves from a narrow, linear approach, (b) become more skilled in identifying the real problems of clients, (c) learn how to address the existential, familial, societal, ethnic, cultural, and spiritual factors that may be associated with the client's suffering, (d) learn how to help clients explore the deeper issues of their lives, (e) develop the personal, interpersonal, and artistic skills needed to deal more effectively with the inherent "messiness" of therapeutic work, and (e) learn how to foster the kind of therapeutic relationship that can bring healing to the troubled client. In short, adopting an overarching HE theoretical framework can help short-term, linear therapists to expand their clinical abilities and become more effective psychotherapists.

If one observed psychotherapy naively (i.e., without knowing anything about the medical model or any other descriptive system), there is almost nothing about the process that would lead one to describe it in medical terms.

Chapter Three

The Medical Model in Psychotherapy: Its Limitations and Failures

Chapter Overview: *The chapter describes the limitations and failures of the medical model by showing that (a) the model does not accurately describe what actually occurs in psychotherapy, (b) the model continues to dominate the field not because of its accuracy but because of its questionable ties with medicine, science, and the health insurance industry, (c) the model obscures the fact that psychotherapy is an interpersonal process, not a medical procedure, and (d) the model fails to account for the fact that thousands of clients use psychotherapy for support, guidance, and personal growth instead of "treatment for mental illness."*

Despite criticism from many psychologists and consumers, the medical model remains the dominant schema for describing clients, their problems, and the process of psychotherapy (Bohart & Tallman, 1999; McCready, 1986; O'Hara, 1996; Szasz, 1974, 1978). In fact, the medical model is so pervasive in mainstream American psychology that, like the fish that had no concept of water, many psychologists have difficulty defining the term. As McCready (1986) wrote:

> What exactly constitutes the "medical model" is difficult to articulate. Certainly there are varying degrees of adherence in practice. However, some general characteristics may be identified. These characteristics in their extreme may include unequivocal subscription to the disease model of emotional disturbance, a paternalistic hierarchy of providers, narrowly

defined treatment parameters, nosological obsessions and nomothetic paradigms. (p. 1)

Bohart and Tallman (1999) raised concerns about the medical model and gave the following overview:

> Psychotherapy originally arose from medicine. Despite efforts to free it from medicine over the years, much of its practice is still heavily influenced by medical-like thinking.... In the medical model, the therapist is analogous to a physician. He or she is the expert on the nature of the client's problems and on how to remediate those problems. He or she forms a diagnosis of the client and then prescribes treatment. Treatment consists of applying interventions appropriate to that diagnosis. These interventions cause change in the client, thereby alleviating the symptom. (p. 5)

Although I find the above descriptions helpful, I would personally define the model as follows: The medical model in psychotherapy is a descriptive schema borrowed from the practice of medicine and superimposed on the practice of psychotherapy. The schema--including its assumptions and terminology--accurately describes the processes and procedures of medical practice and has been highly useful in that field. However, the schema does not accurately describe the processes and procedures of psychotherapy and has proven itself to be problematic when superimposed on that field. In medicine, a doctor diagnoses a patient on the basis of symptoms and administers treatment designed to cure the patient's illness. In psychotherapy, medical model adherents *say* that a doctor diagnoses a patient on the basis of symptoms and administers treatment designed to cure the patient's illness. However, when they say this, they are superimposing a medical schema on psychotherapy and using medical terms to describe what is essentially an interpersonal process that has almost nothing to do with medicine. Thus, the thesis of this chapter is that the superimposition of a medical schema on the nonmedical process of psychotherapy is seriously problematic. Specifically, the chapter will describe the limitations and failures of the medical model in psychotherapy.

A Brief History of the Medical Model in Psychotherapy

The medical model in psychotherapy began with Freud. He was a physician committed to finding a cure for hysteria, a common affliction of women in the Victorian Age (Jones, 1953). In time, Freud developed what Joseph Breuer and his patient "Anna O." had called the "talking cure" (Breuer & Freud, 1893-1895). The new procedure, known as psychoanalysis, was a product of the medical community and everything associated with it was cast in medical terms. Hysteria, along with other psychological problems identified by Freud, was a "mental illness." A "doctor" "diagnosed" the "patient' on the basis of "symptoms" and administered "treatments" designed to "cure" the "illness." Thus, the medical model was applied to psychological problems and psychotherapeutic processes as it had been applied to physical illness and healing.

From the beginning, however, it was obvious that the medical model was problematic. For example, much of what was called "mental illness" was not the same as physical illness. For one thing, patients got better by talking about their "mental illness" whereas talking about one's physical illness had no significant effect. Further, "mental illness," it seemed, was caused by personal and interpersonal difficulties, not by pathogens or physiochemical processes, as was true for physical illness. Also, many psychotherapists sensed a contradiction between the medical model's description of therapy and what actually occurred in therapy. For example, they knew it required a stretch in logic to say that listening to a woman pour out her grief about the loss of a child and offering support was a "medical treatment" or that trying to comfort a man talking about his abject loneliness was a "medical procedure." Nevertheless, the early psychoanalytic community, following the example of Freud, continued to use the medical model as the primary descriptive schema for psychotherapy.

When behaviorism arose in the 1920s under the charismatic leadership of John B. Watson, it enjoyed a great deal of respect and power because it represented a new and exciting explanatory system for what Freudians had called "mental illness" and because behaviorism was associated with science, research, and prestigious academic centers. In the beginning, behaviorism refused to associate itself with the medical model. Indeed, many behaviorists, including

Watson himself, eschewed the medical model, saying that what had been called mental illness was often nothing more than faulty conditioning and learning experiences. In our day, however, the therapeutic offspring of behaviorism have aligned themselves with the medical model. For example, cognitive behavioral therapy (CBT) and certain desensitization treatments, direct therapeutic descendants of behaviorism, are now marketed to managed care and other health insurance companies as "empirically supported treatments" and doctors who specialize in these treatments are reimbursed by medical insurance. Thus, behaviorism, which once boldly rejected the medical model, has now become a major ally of the medical establishment and the health insurance industry.

Humanistic psychology arose as a "third force" in American psychology in the 1950s and 1960s. The human potential movement, the wilder and more popular cousin of humanistic psychology, took humanistic ideals into the streets of America in the form of thousands of workshops, encounter groups, sensitivity training labs, personal growth groups, and various kinds of individual therapeutic experiences (Lieberman, Miles, & Yalom, 1973; Rogers, 1970). During that decade, America became a "therapeutic culture," with literally millions of individuals participating in some form of therapeutic activities (Bellah, Madsen, Sullivan, Swidler, & Tipton, 1985). The vast majority of those who took part in these activities did not view themselves as participating in "treatments for mental illness." Indeed, I suspect this idea seldom, if ever, crossed their minds. The focus of the human potential movement and the "therapeutic culture" of the 1960s was not on curing mental illness but on personal growth, self-awareness, improved relationships, and more effective interpersonal skills (Rogers, 1970).

From the outset, humanistic psychologists were critical of the medical model, seeing it as part of what was wrong with the psychology of the day. As early as the 1940s, Carl Rogers (1951) had begun using the term "clients" instead of "patients" to describe those he saw in therapy. He was also opposed to the use of diagnostic labels and to traditional psychological testing that was designed to discover "pathology." In short, Rogers rejected the medical model and its trappings in favor of a model that viewed therapy as an interpersonal process characterized by empathy, unconditional positive regard, and therapist congruence.

The history of humanistic psychology, however, has not been untainted by involvement with the medical model. Despite the fact that humanistic psychology has always been philosophically opposed to the model, the truth is, many of us "played the medical model game," especially in the 1980s, in order to receive reimbursements from health insurance companies. In 1979, when the U.S. Court of Appeals for the Fourth Circuit in the Commonwealth of Virginia ruled that Blue Shield (and by implication, other health insurance companies) must reimburse psychologists directly for psychological services in the same way they reimbursed psychiatrists, many humanistic clinicians, along with clinicians from other orientations, jumped on the insurance "gravy wagon" and built practices on third party payments. In the 1990s, with the rise of managed care, the chickens came home to roost, so to speak, and we saw the results of having made a bargain with the medical establishment. Clinicians who were dependent on medical insurance reimbursements found it difficult to survive in a managed care world where the number of therapy sessions and the amount of reimbursements were seriously curtailed (see Miller, 1994, 1996a, 1996b, 1996c, for a discussion of managed care rationing and see O'Hara, 1996, for a description of the "bargain" clinicians made with health insurance companies and what was given up in the process). Nevertheless, humanistic psychology-- which includes humanistic, existential, transpersonal, and constructivist approaches--continues to be the dominant voice opposing the medical model. Many counseling psychologists, licensed clinical social workers, and marriage and family therapists-- along with an array of therapists who subscribe to postmodern, feminist, multicultural, and systems approaches--share humanistic psychology's concerns and also stand opposed to the medical model.

Mainstream clinical psychology is permeated by the medical model. Terms such as doctor, patient, symptoms, diagnosis, pathology, mental disorders, and treatments are the "language currency" of the field. The American Psychological Association (APA) is committed to the medical model and even backs prescription privileges for psychologists. As Bohart and Tallman (1999) pointed out, the *APA Monitor*, the organization's monthly news magazine, is filled with articles and advertisements reflecting medical model assumptions. Further, the *Diagnostic and Statistical Manual of Mental Disorders (DSM)*, published by the American

Psychiatric Association (2000), is regarded as the diagnostic "Bible" by thousands of clinical psychologists, with few seeming to question its assumptions or use. Mental illness (or mental disorder) is the accepted term among mainstream clinical psychologists for numerous behaviors and subjective experiences that are problematic or that do not fit the cultural norm. Across America, in hospitals, clinics, and community mental health centers, "doctors" (i.e., psychologists and psychiatrists) "diagnose" the "pathology" of "patients" on the basis of "symptoms" and administer "treatments" in an effort to "cure" "mental disorders." "Empirically supported treatments" (a term suggesting a marriage of science and medicine) is the latest watchword in the long history of the medical model in psychotherapy that stretches from Freud to the present day.

How the Medical Model Maintains
Its Dominance in Psychotherapy

Despite the popularity of the medical model in mainstream clinical psychology, or perhaps because of it, we need to take a critical look at this model. One of the first things we notice is that the typical psychotherapeutic experience, looked at objectively, has almost nothing to do with medicine. It consists of a client who is having some kind of difficulty in life talking with a professional about that difficulty and receiving support, learning skills, or following a regimen that the professional suggests will help mitigate the problem. If one observed psychotherapy naively (i.e., without knowing anything about the medical model or any other descriptive system), there is almost nothing about the process that would lead one to describe it in medical terms. I would suggest one of the main reasons we do so is that historically the schema or "grid" of the medical model was superimposed on the psychotherapeutic process by Freud and others, and for more than a century we have become so accustomed to describing psychotherapy in medical model terms that it is difficult, if not impossible, to remove the medical model "grid" in order to see the process of psychotherapy as it actually is. What confuses things even more (and adds to the difficulty of setting aside the grid) is that *some* mental, emotional, and behavioral problems (e.g., Downs syndrome, autism, Alzheimer's, mental retardation, etc.) *do* have genetic or physiochemical causes. In these cases the medical model *is* the proper descriptive system. Unfortunately, however, this makes it easier to extend the model (almost by sleight-of-hand) to other mental, emotional, and behavioral problems that are not illnesses in any literal sense of the term but are, rather, simply difficult human experiences brought on by faulty learning, inadequate coping skills, stressful events, or other problems in the personal and interpersonal arenas of life. When we label such phenomena "mental illnesses," we are speaking in analogical rather than literal terms.

Unfortunately, many clinicians fail to see that the medical model, when applied to psychotherapy, is an analogical system and that what they call "mental illnesses" are only so in the analogical or metaphorical sense. In other words, they are not illnesses at all in the literal or medical meaning of the term. As psychiatrist Thomas Szasz (1974, 1978) put it--mental illness is a myth. This does not mean that clients do not have real problems or do not experience real emotional pain. Instead, it means that when we label their problems and pain "mental illnesses," we have moved from literal description to analogical description. In other words, we have taken a schema indigenous to medicine and used it as an elaborate analogy to describe psychotherapy. The reason many bright, well-educated clinicians fail to see this is that the medical model lends itself to this kind of confusion, i.e., it lends itself to being taken literally when it is only analogical. Normally, analogies are intended to illumine and clarify, but the medical model, as an analogy, obscures, confuses, and leads even clinicians to believe that certain problems of clients are literally "mental illnesses" when they are not. McCready (1986) suggested we use the term *medical metaphor* instead of *medical model* in order to make the analogical nature of the schema more evident. He wrote:

> *Webster's Dictionary* lists a relevant definition of "model" as: "An example for imitation or emulation." A metaphor, in contrast, is defined as "a figure of speech in which a word or phrase literally denoting one kind of object or idea is used in place of another to suggest a likeness or analogy between them." Thus, the medical model presents psychotherapy as a discipline striving to be like medicine while the medical metaphor depicts psychotherapy as a discipline with its own identity that employs a figure of speech to convey the meaning and benefit of difficult abstract concepts. (p. 3)

It is unlikely, of course, that the psychotherapy profession will adopt McCready's suggestion, but his point is important because it helps us to see that the medical model, when applied to psychotherapy, is a metaphorical rather than a literal system.

If the medical model is so limited and problematic, one must ask: Why does the model remain so dominant in the field of psychotherapy? To answer this question, we must look at the politics of power and economics. It is apparent that the medical model lends a type of status and respectability to psychotherapy because of the model's association with two powerful systems in our culture--medicine and science. When we use terms such as doctor, patient, symptoms, diagnosis, illness, and treatments, we are aligning psychotherapy with medicine, one of the most respected systems in Western culture. Similarly, when we use terms such as "empirically supported treatments" and "evidence based practice," we are aligning psychotherapy with science, the most respected and powerful epistemological system in our culture. Thus, by describing psychotherapy in medical and scientific terms, we create an aura of power and respectability around psychotherapy that is borrowed from these two systems (i.e., medicine and science).

Imagine the loss of prestige that would occur if we described psychotherapy as simply "listening to a person who is demoralized, experiencing emotional pain, or having difficulties in life and giving that person support and guidance based on our experience and psychological knowledge." While such a description is quite accurate in terms of what we actually do, the description lacks the connotations of prestige and power that are associated with saying that we are "doctors engaged in evidence-based practice who diagnose mental disorders and treat patients with empirically supported procedures." The first description conjures up images of a teacher, pastor, counselor, or even a wise friend helping another human being who is having a difficult time. The second description conjures up images of physician-like experts administering medical treatments scientifically proven to cure mental disorders. The power differential in these two descriptive systems is obvious. The first description suggests that psychotherapy is little more than a specialized form of interpersonal relationship. The second suggests that psychotherapy is a medical procedure that has all the power and credibility of medicine and science. The medical model makes what we do sound so prestigious! Add to this the fact that health insurance companies are willing to pay "doctors" for "treating" "mental disorders" but are not willing to pay someone, even a professional with years of training in psychology, to listen to a demoralized person and offer support and guidance, and one can begin to see why the medical model is so entrenched in our profession. *To put it simply, the medical model has remained the dominant descriptive system for psychotherapy, not because it offers the most accurate description of what actually occurs in therapy, but rather because the model's association with medicine and science gives psychotherapy a level of cultural respectability and economic advantages that other descriptive systems do not.* Thus, it will be difficult for any alternative system--regardless how accurate and clinically useful it might be--to replace the medical model because of the powerful political and economic forces that keep the model in place.

Why Psychotherapy Cannot Be Contained
By the Medical Establishment

With all the political and economic power that supports the medical model, it is somewhat puzzling that there has been a historical tendency on the part of psychotherapy to break out of the medical establishment, shed its medical garments, and go running, as it were, into the streets of Western culture. Almost before Freud could say "medical treatment," other pioneers in psychotherapy such as Carl Jung (1912/1956; 1921/1971) and Alfred Adler (1929, 1930, 1931) were already seeing the relevance of psychotherapy to individuation, personal transformation, the education of children, and other areas. In the early 1900s, as psychoanalysis became more widely known and accessible, many individuals went into analysis not because they had a "mental illness" but because the new procedure offered opportunities for greater self-awareness and personal development. For example, Jung saw many midlife patients who had no serious "pathology" but who nevertheless traveled to Switzerland to enter analysis because of Jung's purported wisdom and expertise in helping people to deepen and transform their lives (Brome, 1981; Jung, 1933, 1961). Other early analysts, including Freud himself, saw individuals in therapy who wanted an analysis for personal rather than medical reasons or who wanted to be analyzed so that they could become analysts themselves. Freud even analyzed his own daughter, Anna, as part of her training (Young-Breul, 1988). Thus, while the pioneers in psychotherapy were publishing books, writing articles, and giving professional presentations that described psychotherapy in medical terms such as diagnosis, symptoms, treatments, and cures, they were doing a great deal of therapy that had little or nothing to do with mental illness. In fact, over the past 100 years, and particularly in the second half of the 20th century, it is safe to say that the vast majority of "patients" who entered psychotherapy did so *not* because they were mentally ill but, rather, because of problems in living or because they wanted to use therapy as a vehicle for personal growth. *This fact is almost completely ignored by ardent proponents of the medical model who continue to insist that psychotherapy is a medical treatment for mental disorders.* While psychotherapy has certainly shown itself effective in treating "mental disorders," it is also a culturally-sanctioned way for thousands of people from a large cross-section of American society to avail themselves of personal counsel in times of distress and a way for them to enhance their personal development as human beings. Indeed, as I will discuss in more detail below, the widespread popularity of psychotherapy in our day is due to the fact that Americans know that therapy is not simply a medical procedure for treating mental illness but a process they can use for personal growth and for support and guidance during difficult times. How this revolutionary change in the way psychotherapy is viewed and used in our culture came about is discussed next.[2]

The Psychotherapy Revolution in 20th Century America

In 1985, Robert Bellah, a professor at the University of California, Berkeley, along with his co-authors wrote *Habits of the*

---

[2] I realize, of course, that it's an oversimplification to dichotomize the reasons individuals seek therapy into "problems in living" and "mental illness." For example, it's difficult to know exactly where on the continuum "problems in living" turn into more serious emotional problems. Also, individuals who enter therapy for "personal growth" may discover more serious problems than they had anticipated. Nevertheless, it is still true that the vast majority of psychotherapy clients are there for reasons other than serious "mental illness"--and that's the point I am making here.

Heart: Individualism and Commitment in American Life (1985). The book was a major sociological analysis of American culture and was immediately hailed as a landmark study. Bellah, along with his four co-authors, named the rise of a "therapeutic culture" in America one of the major trends of the 20th century. He said that widespread use of psychotherapy arose in response to the fragmentation of relationships that came as a result of the rise of national occupations that required individuals to move away from small towns and communities where they had grown up. Whereas one's profession had once been a way to ensure one's unique place in the social and economic fabric of a small community, in the 1800s this began to change so that by the 1900s many individuals were pursuing occupations that required them to leave their communities and move to large urban areas. What was important for many in this new occupational world was the ability to quickly form relationships and then leave them behind as they moved up the corporate ladder and across the nation. In this cultural situation, psychotherapy arose as both an analogue of society's quick and time-limited relationships as well as a "training ground" in which one could learn to function more effectively in the fragmented society of individualism. Further, the therapeutic relationship supplied the support and guidance that traditional relationships had once supplied in families and small towns. Thus, while psychotherapy had been conceptualized originally by Freud and others as a medical treatment for mental illness, it became, in the 20th century, a cultural phenomenon that arose to address the psychic needs of individuals subjected to the "new world" where community and traditional relationships were abrogated. As Bellah et al. (1985) said:

> It is in this context that we should interpret the emergence of the therapeutic culture and therapeutic relationships that became ever more important in the twentieth century. Such therapy was probably more a support for those placed under unprecedented psychic demands than a cure for new mental ills. (p. 119)

Bellah et al. went on to say that "the support that traditional relationships no longer adequately supplied to the overburdened individual now came in the form of new institutions" (p. 121). Psychotherapy was one of those "new institutions." Bellah et al.

insightfully noted that psychotherapy consisted of "a relationship between a patient (or client) and a professional therapist" and that "this relationship is itself the chief instrument of the therapy" (p. 121). Psychotherapy grew into a major cultural force in the second half of the 20th century. Bellah et al. (1985) said:

> While we have no accurate statistics on the number of people using psychotherapy in twentieth-century America, there is reason to believe that there has been a steady increase, particularly since World War II, with three times as many Americans seeing "mental health professionals" now as did twenty years ago. Young, urban, well-educated people from professional backgrounds are the most likely to have actually sought professional therapeutic help, but by 1976 all sections of society turned more frequently to professional care. (p. 121)

This analysis by Bellah et al. makes it clear that psychotherapy did not expand because it was a medical treatment for mental illness but, rather, because it offered a supportive relationship to those who were experiencing difficulties associated with the loss of community and traditional relationships in American culture. When the large-scale growth of psychotherapy is viewed from this meta-perspective, it becomes obvious that proponents of the medical model who continue to insist that psychotherapy is a treatment for mental illness are out of touch with what is actually happening to psychotherapy in American society. *This constitutes yet another major limitation of the medical model: the model cannot account for the fact that the vast majority of clients in psychotherapy are there for reasons other than mental illness.*

Summary and Implications

To summarize, the medical model has serious limitations: (a) the model fails to describe accurately what actually occurs in therapy; (b) the model continues to dominate the field not because of its accuracy but rather because of its questionable ties with medicine, science, and the health insurance industry; (c) the model obscures the fact that psychotherapy is primarily an interpersonal process rather than a medical procedure; and (d) the model cannot account for the fact that the vast majority of clients who seek psychotherapy do so for reasons other than mental illness.

The analysis of the medical model presented in this chapter has important implications. First, we must decide what our posture will be relative to the medical model. Making this decision is not easy. If we disavow the medical model, we take ourselves out of the mainstream and make ourselves vulnerable to political and economic repercussions from the forces that keep the model in place. Also, the model is so ingrained in our clinics, training programs, research centers, and professional organizations that it is difficult to reject it even if we would like to do so. On the other hand, if we decide to embrace the model we are thereby giving our support to an inaccurate and problematic system that may cause harm to clients and create other ethical problems. Thus, we are caught in a dilemma that motivates some to seek a middle ground such as continuing to expose the limitations and failures of the medical model while making accommodations, when necessary, to the reality of the model's pervasiveness in the profession. Thus, we have three basic choices: (a) reject the medical model, (b) embrace the model, or (c) try to find some middle ground. Because the model is so problematic and yet pervasive, any course we choose will have its own set of problems.

Second, we must consider the ethical implications of diagnosing clients with a "mental disorder" when a more accurate model would suggest that those clients are simply reacting in a human way to the difficulties of life. To put it another way, do we have the right to label human beings with a "mental disorder" when a more accurate model would suggest that they are not "mentally disordered" at all? The following example is one to which even ardent proponents of the medical model can relate. In its discussion of bereaved clients, the *DSM* indicates that symptoms of depression are normal for those who have lost a loved one. But then the *DSM* says that if those symptoms persist for more than two months, the client should be diagnosed as clinically depressed. To make this less abstract, imagine an older woman who comes to therapy because she has lost her life-long mate. Two months have passed and she is still having a difficult time--as anybody with half a heart would understand. Would any humane clinician really conclude that this woman has a "mental disorder" simply because she is still grieving the loss of a mate with whom she has spent her entire adult life? What kind of profession--

and what kind of model of psychotherapy--would come to such an inhumane conclusion? As I tell my graduate students, it takes me two months to get over a stumped toe and the DSM wants me to get over the loss of a loved one in that same length of time! As my students might say, "What's wrong with this picture?" Admittedly, this is a dramatic example, but I believe it shows just how easily a normal person reacting in a normal way can be diagnosed with a "mental disorder." Can we be ethical human beings and participate in this kind of inhumaneness?

Third, we must ask ourselves about the ethical implications of collaborating with managed care and other health insurance companies in certain ways. For example, is it ethical to reveal diagnoses and other personal information about our clients in order to persuade insurance companies to reimburse our services? This is an old question with which many of us have struggled since the time insurance companies, and particularly managed care, began demanding more information about clients before reimbursing psychotherapists. Relatedly, is it ethical to terminate psychotherapy with clients against our better clinical judgment just because a managed care company insists on rationing the number of sessions for economic reasons. These are serious ethical issues that have to do with the welfare of clients. Such issues arise because our profession is so dependent on, and entangled with, the medical model and the health insurance industry.

Fourth, we must ask ourselves about the ethical implications of "playing the medical model game" and "pushing the diagnostic envelope" by giving clients diagnoses whose treatments are reimbursable by medical insurance if we know in our hearts that those clients are just as sane and normal as we are. If we know better but play the game anyway, are we prostituting ourselves for economic gain? It is a hard question but one worthy of careful consideration.

Fifth, we must reevaluate our use of such tools as the *DSM*. Clearly, the *DSM* contains helpful descriptions of certain configurations of mental, emotional, and behavioral problems. In that regard, the *DSM* is a useful reference to help students and clinicians to recognize problematic patterns in clients' lives that might otherwise be overlooked. If the *DSM* stopped at the descriptive level, it would be an excellent resource not subject to serious criticism. However, the *DSM*, as a tool of the medical model, goes further by saying that these patterns are "diagnostic categories" and "mental disorders." There is no apparent reason for the *DSM* to move from description to diagnosis except that by doing so, the *DSM* remains true to its medical model origins and serves as a powerful, legitimizing tool to persuade health insurance companies to pay for treatments. In other words, by taking the additional step of turning descriptive patterns into "diagnoses" and "mental disorders," the *DSM* legitimizes the "treatment" of those "disorders" and, of course, reimbursements of the "doctor" by medical insurance. Once again, we see just how entangled the medical model is with economics.

Sixth, if the analysis presented in this chapter is correct, we should "own" what we do in psychotherapy. For example, if we work with patients who are truly mentally ill, meaning their problems are due to genetic or physiochemical processes gone awry, then perhaps we have a right to say that we treat mental illness. However, if we work primarily with clients who are in therapy for support and guidance as they struggle with the difficulties of life, then we have an obligation, it seems to me, to "own" that this is what we are doing instead of "treating mental disorders." Unfortunately, some of us experience a type of "professional guilt" when we admit that we are seeing clients who are not mentally ill but who are struggling with problems in living or who have come to therapy to enhance their personal development. This seems strange. Teachers don't feel guilty for teaching healthy students. Pastors and rabbis don't feel guilty for providing guidance to healthy parishioners. Yet, when it comes to psychotherapists, some of us have an uneasy feeling that there's something wrong, or at least not quite right, with making therapy available to those who are not mentally ill. I would suggest that this sense of "professional guilt" is due to the power and influence of the medical model over our own psyches. The "guilt mantra" goes something like this: "Psychotherapy is a treatment for the mentally ill, so if you use it to help people who are not mentally ill, you are misusing this medical treatment on people who don't really need it." Some, it seems, have accepted this mantra without really examining it.

Certainly, it is important for us to ask ourselves where we, with our particular constellation of abilities, can most effectively serve. This kind of self-reflection will lead some to dedicate their lives to serving those with severe mental difficulties. Some will even decide to work on the "back wards" of mental hospitals or in prisons for the criminally insane where they will try to bring some measure of help and comfort to those who suffer the horrors of severe mental and emotional disturbances. Clinicians who choose to work in such difficult venues deserve our respect and admiration. Others of us, however, will realize that we are not cut out for that kind of work and that, if we forced ourselves to do it, we would either burn out quickly or become depressed or go insane (and I mean that quite literally). However, we *can* dedicate our lives to helping those who are struggling with stress, anxiety, depression, ennui, and other personal and interpersonal problems associated with living in today's world. *This kind of work can be just as honorable as working with those who are seriously mentally and emotionally impaired.*

If we help a woman who is being abused by her husband so that she takes herself and her children out of harm's way and eventually constructs a better life, who can measure the importance of that? If we help a father and mother to stop verbally abusing their children and show them a better way to parent, who can measure the positive effects on those children and perhaps even on future generations of that family? If we talk to a teenage girl who wants to die because she feels that no one cares or understands and if our support prevents her from killing herself so that she goes on to create a meaningful life, who can measure that? If we talk to a lonely old man who feels nobody appreciates the life he lived and if we affirm him for what he is and was, who can put a price on the peace he may experience in his final days? *The point is this: it is honorable to help those who are struggling with the difficult problems of life or who come to therapy because they want to become better human beings. There is so much pain and lostness in the world that we should never denigrate those who dedicate their lives to giving comfort, support, and guidance.* It is very telling that in our capitalistic society almost no one raises ethical or moral questions about dedicating one's life to a corporation whose only real goal is the "bottom line." In light of our moral lacunae when it comes to capitalistic pursuits, it seems to me that no one (including ourselves) should ever feel guilty for dedicating his or her life to helping others, regardless what form that dedication takes.

Conclusion: A Radical Proposal

For trainees and clinicians who have no desire to spend their professional lives "playing the game" whose rules are set by the medical model and the health insurance industry, there may be other options. It is worth recalling that historically psychotherapy was not dependent on medical insurance. Although the situation is different today and some would argue that it is impossible to maintain a psychotherapy practice without taking insurance reimbursements, there is reason to believe that many consumers would gladly pay for therapeutic services that are divorced from the diagnosing and pathologizing requirements of the medical model and the invasive demands of the health insurance industry. O'Hara (1996) said:

> There is ample evidence to back the argument that people in our troubled age will want the services of specifically nonmedical therapists or counselors more than ever. Just because managed care has eliminated from the category of "medical necessity" all the ordinary, yet often wrenching, difficulties that may accompany normal life issues and transitions in late 20th century America childhood; peer relationships and schooling; adolescence and leaving home (or not leaving home); courtship; marriage and divorce; childbirth and parenting; work and career; midlife; aging and death--doesn't mean that they will cease to exist. (p. 48)

In 1998, in an article published in the *Journal of the American Medical Association (JAMA)* Eisenberg, Davis, Ettner, Appel, Wilkey, Van Rompay, and Kessler (1998) reported the results of their 1997 survey on alternative therapies. From 1990 (the date of the most recent survey prior to theirs) to 1997 there was a 47.3% increase in total visits to alternative practitioners, from 427 million visits in 1990 to 629 million visits in 1997. *This exceeded total visits to all U.S. primary care physicians!* In 1997, the out-of-pocket expenditures for alternative therapies were conservatively estimated at $27 billion, which was about the same as out-of-pocket expenditures for services from U.S. physicians. Alternative therapies that increased the most from 1990 to 1997 included herbal medicine, massage, megavitamins, self-help groups, folk remedies, energy healing, and homeopathy. The most frequent focus of alternative therapies was chronic conditions such as back problems, anxiety, depression, and headaches.

These findings may have implications for those interested in offering nonmedical psychotherapy services (i.e., services not based on the medical model and not reimbursed by health insurance). It is particularly noteworthy that anxiety and depression, the two leading "mental disorders" in the United States, are often the focus of alternative therapies. Psychotherapists are especially qualified to assist individuals suffering from these problems.

Thus, it seems millions of American consumers are willing to pay billions of dollars in out-of-pocket expenses for alternative therapeutic services. At the same time, there are literally thousands of psychotherapists who would like to practice outside the medical model and without the interference of managed care and the health insurance industry. If bridges could be built that would bring these consumers and therapists together, the results could be quite astounding. Not only would millions of Americans receive competent psychotherapy services for their emotional difficulties, but psychotherapists would be able to free themselves from the stranglehold of the medical establishment and the health insurance industry.

Realistically, the only psychotherapists who could break away from the medical model--at least in the beginning--are private practitioners. For example, it would be almost impossible for therapists who work in hospitals, community mental health centers, and other settings that receive "health care" funding to take such a radical step. And even private practitioners would have a difficult time. If they truly disengaged from the medical model, they would have to give up insurance reimbursements and charge fees, hopefully adjusting those fees (or even doing pro bono work) for clients unable to afford them. To support such a practice, clinicians might have to find creative ways to supplement their income such as college teaching, presenting workshops, or doing other professional work. Some might be fortunate enough to find philanthropic individuals or organizations willing to support their efforts, especially if those efforts focused on special problems or populations. Regardless, those who decide to practice outside the medical and insurance establishment will face many challenges and it is unlikely that they will be as financially secure as those who remain in the system.

That's the bad news. The good news is that there may be other, more important, rewards. As O'Hara (1996) put it,

> The age-old idea of work as something akin to a sacred calling, a vocation inspired by a desire to serve humanity, drives many therapists who choose to buck the tide of managed care yet still want to be in private practice. Another powerful moral incentive is their determination to remain free and independent. Certainly, the ideal of service is more compelling than any hopes of getting rich. It is an ideal that these clinicians often believe has been misplaced by the therapeutic community over the last decade or two. (p. 51)

It is radical to suggest that the best way to deal with the medical model is to reject it completely. However, in our day, psychotherapy is under unprecedented attack by political and economic forces. The medical establishment has little respect for what we do and the health insurance industry would like nothing better than to turn psychotherapy into a "quick-fix" center owned by Wall Street or replace it with an inexpensive pill. Personally, I am concerned about what will happen if we simply "stay the course" and continue to hope that someday the medical establishment and the health insurance industry will give our profession the status and parity it deserves. Despite a few gains now and then by psychotherapists, the most likely scenario is that the medical establishment and the health insurance industry will increasingly marginalize, ration, and reduce psychotherapy until it becomes nothing but a small room in the medical-insurance complex. If we knew that this would be our future, what effect would it have on our thinking and actions today? This is a question worthy of careful reflection.

It may be time for humanistic psychologists to start another revolution in psychology. This time the revolution would involve rejecting the medical model, breaking away from the medical establishment, and telling managed care and the health insurance industry that we will no longer require their services. I realize that humanistic psychology does not have the power to persuade mainstream psychology to follow this path. In fact, because mainstream clinical psychology is so entangled with medicine and insurance, I suspect the revolution would have to focus on breaking away from the mainstream and offering an alternative system of care. Although some would call this an impossible dream, I believe this may be the most opportune time in the history of psychology to consider progressive alternatives. Science has now undermined the medical model and increasing numbers of clinicians and researchers are realizing that we must construct a new approach to psychotherapy. Also, as noted above, there are powerful underground rumblings to suggest that millions of consumers and thousands of psychotherapists are unhappy with the medical model and the health insurance industry. If we were able to tap this frustration, we might be able to establish an alternative system of therapeutic services. Of course, such a revolution would take time, and I have no doubt that, if we broke away from the medical-insurance establishment, we would suffer political and economic repercussions as well as many logistical difficulties. Nevertheless, if we want to save psychotherapy from increasing medicalization and continue to offer the kind of therapeutic services that humanistic practitioners have always offered, we may have no choice but to move in more radical directions.

I have often wondered what it would be like to practice without the interference of the medical model and the insurance companies. Financially, I'm sure it would be difficult, at least in the beginning, but there might be other important rewards. For example, we might go home at night knowing that we had served our clients well and that we had made our own contribution toward eliminating a model that has little to do with what actually occurs in therapy, that is held in place by questionable entanglements with medicine and insurance, that refuses to recognize that psychotherapy is an interpersonal process instead of a medical procedure, and that tends to brand individuals with the stigma of mental illness and diagnostic labels. We might sleep a little better at night, feel more in charge of our own professional lives, and have more passion and excitement about going to work each day. All in all, that would not be such a bad life.

Science has now shown in a clear and convincing way that while psychotherapy is highly effective, no therapeutic modality is any more effective than any other therapeutic modality and no therapeutic techniques are any more effective than any other therapeutic techniques. Instead, therapeutic effectiveness is due to certain other factors in the therapeutic situation that are common to all therapeutic systems. These findings deconstruct, in a devastating way, the whole notion of "empirically supported treatments."

Chapter Four

Empirically Supported Treatments
The Deconstruction of a Myth

Chapter Overview: This chapter summarizes recent findings from analyses and meta-analyses of psychotherapy research which show that so-called empirically supported treatments: (ESTs) are no more effective than traditional psychotherapies, that specific modalities and techniques have little to do with therapeutic effectiveness, and that contextual factors are the major determinants of therapeutic outcome. These scientific findings deconstruct the whole notion of ESTs and make the current debate about them meaningless.

I am not being overly dramatic when I say that our profession is currently engaged in a debate whose outcome may very well determine the future of psychotherapy in America. The debate is about the use of "empirically supported treatments" (ESTs) versus what I will refer to in this chapter as "traditional psychotherapies." Lists of ESTs are dominated by short-term, technique-focused treatments such as behavioral and cognitive behavioral therapy (CBT). "Traditional psychotherapies," as I use the term here, refers to therapies that are generally longer-term, more complex, and less technique-focused such as humanistic, existential, psychodynamic, and systems approaches.

The reason this debate is so important is that it is not simply about which therapeutic approach is "better" or which might be more effective with a particular client or disorder. Our profession has debated these kinds of issues for years, and if that's all the debate were about, there would be no reason for concern. This debate, however, is different and the outcome has enormous implications for the future of psychotherapy. *Let me put it bluntly: the debate is about the complete eradication of all therapeutic approaches that do not meet the so-called "scientific" standards set up by proponents of ESTs.* While not every clinician who uses ESTs endorses such an extreme goal, the more ardent supporters of ESTs believe that all "unscientific" psychotherapies should be abolished and replaced with approaches that are deemed to be "empirically supported." Indeed, some proponents of ESTs (Lohr, Fowler, & Lilienfeld, 2002) have gone so far as to suggest that the American Psychological Association (APA) and other psychology associations should enforce the use of ESTs and "impose stiff sanctions, including expulsion if necessary" (p. 8) against clinicians who do not comply.

So far, APA has refused to take such an extreme position. It is unsettling, however, that APA (2002) now specifically requires, as part of its official accreditation criteria, that psychology programs provide training in ESTs. Clearly, training programs seeking initial or renewed accreditation will view this as an endorsement of ESTs by APA and most will do whatever is necessary to make sure their students receive such training. As this chapter will show, there is no scientific basis for this requirement and APA has clearly gone beyond the evidence to burden programs with this questionable requirement. On the other side of the coin, in 2005, under the leadership of Ronald Levant as APA president, the APA Council of Representatives approved the policy statement of the APA Presidential Task Force on Evidence-Based Practice (2006) which represented a more moderate position on the use of ESTs. (This is discussed later in this chapter). Nevertheless, APA remains a "house divided"--especially at the Division and at individual member levels -- over the issue of the use of ESTs in psychotherapy.

Politics and Elitist Attitudes Cloud the Scientific Issues

Despite all the talk about scientific versus unscientific treatments, this debate is not simply about science. If it were, those of us who support traditional psychotherapies would have nothing to worry about because since the late 1970s and early 1980s the research has clearly shown that psychotherapy, including traditional approaches, is robustly effective (Bergin & Lambert, 1978; Lambert & Bergin, 1994; Lipsey & Wilson 1993; Seligman, 1995; Smith & Glass, 1977; Smith, Glass, & Miller, 1980; Wampold, 2001). In light of this well-established scientific fact, one has to wonder why ardent proponents of ESTs are so critical of traditional psychotherapies and want to replace them with ESTs. The answer, no doubt, is that this debate is not only about science but also about politics, economics, the medical model, managed care, and getting a piece of the health insurance pie. These political and economic matters cloud the scientific issues and ultimately may have more to do with the outcome of the debate than the scientific findings. Thus, it would be naïve for those of us who support traditional psychotherapies to assume that all we have to do is demonstrate the scientific validity of our approaches, and the debate would be over. In fact, we have already done that, and it is had no detectable effect on the debate. The truth is, if we want to win this debate we must be politically sophisticated as well as scientifically grounded.

Ronald Levant (2004), the former president of APA mentioned above, described the attitudes one often encounters when trying to discuss ESTs with ardent supporters. Levant said:

> Empirically-validated treatment is a difficult topic for a practitioner to discuss with clinical scientists. In my attempts to discuss this informally, I have found that some clinical scientists immediately assume that I am anti-science, and others emit a guffaw, asking incredulously: "What, are you for empirically *unsupported* treatments?" McFall (1991, p. 76) reflects this perspective when he divides the world of clinical psychology into "scientific and pseudoscientific clinical psychology," and rhetorically asks "what is the alternative [to

scientific   clinical   psychology]?   *Unscientific*   clinical
psychology" (See also Lilienfeld, Lohr, & Morier, 2001).

There are, thus, some ardent clinical scientists... who
appear to subscribe to scientistic faith and believe that the
superiority of scientific approach is so marked that other
approaches should be excluded. Since this is a matter of faith
rather than reason, arguments would seem to be pointless....
Punctuating   these   interactions   from   the   practitioner
perspective, the controversy seems to stem from the attempts
of some clinical scientists to dominate the discourse on
acceptable practice, and impose very narrow views of both
science and practice. (p. 219)

Unfortunately, the elitist attitudes that Levant describes are
part of the political realities of this debate. The history of psychology
is rife with examples of those who were so sure of their own
"scientific" views that they marginalized those who disagreed with
them. Freud started it by banishing such luminaries as Carl Jung and
Alfred Adler from his inner circle. John Watson (Watson & Raynor,
1920) continued the trend in the early 1900s by touting the
"scientific" basis of behaviorism and publicly taunting psychoanalysts
(after he had psychologically abused "Little Albert"). Today, such
elitist attitudes characterize those who, in the name of "science,"
would eliminate all therapeutic approaches except their own. While
we must be tolerant, as William James put it, toward those who
themselves are tolerant, we must challenge colleagues who insist that
they have a monopoly on therapeutic truth and who would, if they had
their way, eliminate all therapeutic modalities except those they deem
to be "empirically supported." It is also important that we monitor our
own motives and remember that this debate is not about our own
egos, or even, ultimately, about our own professional futures.
Something much larger is at stake. *This debate is about the future of
psychotherapy as a healing art and about the thousands of clients,
present and future, who desperately need the kind of therapeutic
experience that traditional psychotherapies provide* (see Elkins,
2008; Miller, 1994, 1996a,1996b, 1996c; and Seligman, 1995, for
information on the benefits of longer-term therapy). The stakes in this
debate could not be higher. It is a debate we cannot afford to lose.

Empirically Supported Treatments: A Brief History

In the late 1970s, psychology began to put "all of the eggs in the 'technique' basket" (Bergin, 1997, p. 83). In the 1980s, managed care companies and the health insurance industry in general put pressure on psychology to demonstrate that it could do both efficient and effective psychotherapy. In keeping with their medical model assumptions, the companies wanted psychology to identify specific treatments that were scientifically proven to be effective for specific disorders. In 1993, responding to the pressure and wanting to ensure that psychologists got a piece of the health insurance pie, Division 12, Society of Clinical Psychology, of APA, formed a task force to identify effective therapies and publicize these to psychologists, health insurance companies, and the public. The task force created a list of treatments which they referred to as "well-established" and "probably efficacious" (Task Force on Promotion and Dissemination of Psychological Procedures, 1995, p. 3). In time, the terminology was changed to "empirically validated treatments" (EVTs) and later, to "empirically supported treatments." The Division 12 list of ESTs was dominated by short-term behavioral and cognitive-behavioral treatments. Traditional psychotherapies, which tend to be longer-term, more complex, and less technique-focused, did not make the list. By creating and publishing their list of ESTs, the Division 12 task force joined with managed care and health insurance companies in taking psychotherapy down a road that many of us in humanistic psychology feared would be the end of psychotherapy as we had known it. When the task force made it clear that ESTs must be administered using manualized instructions, we were even more disturbed. Then, when the task force urged APA to make adherence to ESTs a major criterion for accreditation and even for approving continuing education sponsors, some of us were about ready to throw in the towel. Then, when it was rumored that clinicians who failed to use ESTs would be vulnerable to charges of professional incompetence and unethical practice and could be sued by clients for not meeting "standard of care" requirements, we became nauseous and fell into existential despair. Finally, when some proponents of ESTs, apparently getting into the spirit of things a bit too much, went so far as to say that APA should enforce the use of ESTs and sanction or expel those who refused to comply, many of us concluded the apocalypse was here and the end of the world was at hand. Those of us with weak ego strength and paranoid tendencies were haunted by visions of being lined up against clinic walls or in university commons and shot for having humanistic or existential inclinations. The more reality-oriented ones among us envisioned a managed care world where technician-like therapists, manuals in hand, would administer ESTs to treat depression, panic, phobias, generalized anxiety disorder, and other emotional problems using the short-term formats demanded by managed care and enforced by its checklist-using clerks. A few humanistic clinicians, perhaps panicked about their economic futures, began offering workshops on short-term therapy, trying to show that we, too, could fit into the new managed care world. Others, believing in the basic scientific soundness of humanistic therapies, criticized traditional research methods and called, with little success, for the inclusion of qualitative approaches in determining what treatments would be deemed empirically supported.

Fortunately, when Division 12's list of ESTs was made public, there was "an attendant landslide of criticism from practitioners and researchers who found the project to be scientifically questionable as well as overzealous in its assertions" (Lambert & Barley, 2002, p. 17). Division 32, Society for Humanistic Psychology, along with other APA divisions, voiced strong concerns about the direction of the Division 12 task force and succeeded in getting individuals on the committee who were able to moderate, at least to a degree, some of the committee's more extreme goals. Division 32 formed a task force of its own (Task Force for the Development of Guidelines for the Provision of Humanistic Psychosocial Services, 1997) to establish humanistic guidelines and to offer an alternative to those proposed by the Division 12 task force. Division 17, Society of Counseling Psychology, also got into the act and issued principles that challenged Division 12's methods for determining empirically supported approaches (Wampold, Lichtenberg, & Waehler, 2002). Division 29, Division of Psychotherapy, also established a task force (Task Force on Empirically-Supported Therapy Relationships) to identify and publish the scientific evidence showing that the therapeutic relationship is a major determinant of therapeutic outcome, thus counterbalancing Division 12's emphasis on "empirically supported treatments" (ESTs) with what the Division 29 task force called "empirically supported relationships" (ESRs). (See Norcross, 2001, 2002, for a comprehensive presentation of the work of the Division 29 task force).

The general outcry from researchers and clinicians, along with the actions of Division 32, Division 17, Division 29, and other APA divisions had an effect. Indeed, those efforts may have saved psychotherapy, at least for the time being, from being redefined as a short-term, manualized, technique-dominated enterprise. To date, neither Division 12 nor APA has mandated the exclusive use of ESTs and, to my knowledge, no clinicians have been shot, sued, sanctioned, kicked out of APA, or charged with professional incompetence or unethical conduct for refusing to follow the official list of ESTs. In fact, as noted earlier, when clinician Ronald Levant was president of APA in 2005, he commissioned a task force on evidence-based practice in psychology (EBPP). The APA Presidential Task Force on Evidence-Based Practice (2006), as the committee was called, issued a policy statement on evidence-based practice that was approved by the APA Council of Representatives. The report of the task force, which was published in the *American Psychologist* (APA Presidential Task Force on Evidence-Based Practice, 2006), makes it clear that EBPP is a broader concept than ESTs, giving psychologists greater leeway in using clinical expertise to determine which treatments are best for a particular client and how, considering all research evidence, to adapt treatments to individual situations. The task force defined EBPP as follows: "*Evidence-based practice in psychology* (EBPP) is the integration of the best available research with clinical expertise in the context of patient characteristics, culture, and preferences" (*APA Presidential Task Force on Evidence-Based Practice in Psychology*, 2006, p. 273). This report, which represents APA's current position, is clearly a more moderate posture than the extreme position taken by the original task force of Division 12. Thus, a battle was won, at least in part, for those of us who believed in the effectiveness of traditional psychotherapies and who did not endorse the exclusive use of ESTs.

Why Traditional Psychotherapies Are in Danger

We must not, however, think the conflict is over. While we may have won a battle, we are still in grave danger of losing the war. Many psychologists believe the Division 12 task force was right to advocate the use of ESTs. Many graduate training programs, internship sites, and mental health clinics endorse the use of ESTs. Managed care and the health insurance industry in general, along with governmental agencies and research centers, still believe that ESTs are the only way to go. Many professors and clinical supervisors in graduate training programs tell students that competent treatment can only be delivered by using ESTs. Perhaps most disturbing of all, as noted earlier, the American Psychological Association (2002), in its *Guidelines and Principles for Accreditation of Programs in Professional Psychology*, prescribed competencies in ESTs. The guidelines specifically mentioned that students should receive such training in programs (p. 9), practicum experiences (p. 10), and internships (p. 17). As Wampold (2001) said:

> Although there is no scientific evidence that training should place emphasis on ESTs, the Guidelines and Principles of Accreditation prescribe competencies in ESTs. For example, the Guidelines and Principles for internship sites states that "all interns (should) demonstrate an intermediate to advanced knowledge of professional skills, abilities, proficiencies, competencies, and knowledge in the area of theories and methods of... effective interventions (*including empirically supported treatments*)." (p. 230)

In this milieu, psychology students who are interested in traditional psychotherapies are at a woeful disadvantage. When professors and clinical supervisors tell students that certain approaches, such as CBT, are "empirically based" and that others are merely "theoretical and speculative," it becomes difficult for students to remain committed to therapies not endorsed by their mentors. Because today's psychology students will be the clinicians of tomorrow, there is reason to believe that psychotherapy will be increasingly dominated by therapists who practice CBT and other such "empirically based" approaches. If this occurs, the extreme goals of the Division 12 task force will be realized after all, through an influx of thousands of new clinicians who are committed to ESTs and who, in time, will replace those of us who are practicing today.

Meanwhile, those of us who are committed to traditional psychotherapies look for effective ways to respond to students and others who ask about the scientific bases of our approaches. As this chapter will show, some scholars among us are able to reframe the issue and provide very clear and convincing answers. Most of us, however, tend to respond in one or more of the following ways. First, because we, too, respect science, we sometimes say that our therapeutic approach, while perhaps not scientifically proven, is nevertheless supported by softer forms of "clinical evidence" and many years of "clinical experience." Second, we may launch into a short lecture about the limitations of traditional research methods, implying that if qualitative methods were used, our approach undoubtedly would do well. Third, if we happen to practice from the Person-Centered Approach, we may dust off some of the old research by Carl Rogers and his associates that showed the scientific validity of his "necessary and sufficient" conditions of psychotherapy (of course, this may not do much for those of us who practice from existential, psychodynamic, and systems approaches). Fourth, as a last resort, we may respond that our therapeutic approach is merely "untested," implying that if we ever get around to testing it, it will surely prove to be just as scientific as those that are said to be empirically based.

While such responses have some validity and may be persuasive to the "choir," they are not very convincing to graduate students and others who are already wavering in their commitment to "theoretical and speculative" approaches in favor of those that are said to be scientific and empirically based. Perhaps these arguments had some merit in the 1990s when we were forced to debate managed care and the Division 12 task force about which modalities and techniques were "empirically supported." *Today, however, I believe these arguments are inadequate and misguided. The problem with all the arguments is that they are based on the assumption that we should be able to demonstrate scientifically that our particular modality and techniques produce client improvement and successful therapeutic outcome. As I will show in this chapter, this assumption is problematic, not only because it focuses on the wrong factors in psychotherapy (i.e., modalities and techniques), but also because, from a political and strategic perspective, if we continue to fight the war for traditional psychotherapy on the battleground this assumption created, we will lose.* Admittedly, in the 1990s this was the battleground staked out by managed care and the Division 12 task force, and we had little choice but to fight on their turf and according to their terms. Indeed, some of our colleagues did an excellent job of presenting the research evidence for humanistic therapies, as well as making the case for alternative research approaches in determining the effectiveness of treatments (e.g., Cain & Seeman, 2002; Elliott, 2002; Elliott, Greenberg, & Lietaier, 2003); Task Force for the Development of Practice Recommendations for the Provision of Humanistic Psychosocial Services, 2004). But today things are different and we must shift the debate to a new venue, one created by recent analyses and meta-analyses of the research on therapeutic effectiveness which show what is actually responsible for client improvement and therapeutic outcome (hint: it's *not* modalities and techniques). By shifting the scientific debate to this new venue, we will not only deconstruct the myth of ESTs but we will also demonstrate the scientific validity of our own "theoretical and speculative" approaches to psychotherapy.

Deconstructing ESTs: The Scientific Evidence

One of the remarkable things about science is that it cuts both ways. For example, if a group insists that science and science alone should decide which psychotherapies are effective, that group then has a logical obligation to accept whatever science reveals. *In that regard, science has now shown in a clear and convincing way that while psychotherapy is highly effective, no therapeutic modality is any more effective than any other therapeutic modality and no therapeutic techniques are any more effective than any other therapeutic techniques. Instead, therapeutic effectiveness is due to certain other factors in the therapeutic situation that are common to all therapeutic systems.* As I will show, these findings deconstruct, in a devastating way, the whole notion of "empirically supported treatments" (ESTs). The scientific evidence for these statements is summarized below.

In a landmark study, professor and psychologist Bruce Wampold (2001), chair of the Department of Counseling Psychology at the University of Wisconsin at Madison, who is also a mathematician and statistician, reviewed decades of research and conducted analyses and meta-analyses of thousands of studies in an effort to clarify the determinants of therapeutic effectiveness.

Wampold reported his findings in journal articles (e.g., Ahn Wampold, 1997; Messer & Wampold, 2000; Waehler, Kalodner, Lichtenberg, & Wampold, 2000; Wampold et al., 1997; Wampold, 2001). While other scholars, including Castonguay (1993), Frank and Frank (1991), Grencavage and Norcross (1990), Hubble et al. (1999), Luborsky et al. (1975), Norcross (2001; 2002), Orlinsky, Grave, and Parks (1994), and Rosenweig (1936) and have come to similar conclusions, I will focus on Wampold's book because in my opinion it is the most comprehensive, detailed, and balanced presentation of the scientific evidence relative to the issues addressed in this chapter.[3]

The "debate" referred to in the title of Wampold's (2001) book *The Great Psychotherapy Debate* is the debate over *why* and *how* psychotherapy works. *That* therapy works is no longer a question in the research literature. As noted earlier, since the late 1970s and early 1980s, we have known that psychotherapy is highly effective. But *why* psychotherapy works and *how* it works are questions over which there is still much debate.

As Wampold pointed out, there are two sides to this debate. One side, the *medical model,* says that therapy works because of "specific ingredients," i.e., specific techniques. Thus, for example, proponents of the medical model would say that CBT alleviates clinical depression because of the "specific ingredients" in CBT, meaning the techniques such as challenging negative thoughts which are hypothesized to be maintaining the depression. Thus, the medical model supports the search for specific psychotherapy techniques that will cure specific mental disorders, in much the same way that medical researchers search for specific medications that will cure specific physical illnesses. For obvious reasons, ESTs are the "superstars" of the medical model in psychotherapy.

The other side of the debate, which Wampold called the *contextual model*, argues that it is *not* techniques that are responsible for therapeutic benefits but certain other factors in the therapeutic situation that are common to all therapeutic systems. Wampold (2001) named this the contextual model "because it emphasizes the

---

[3] Many others have also recognized the importance of Wampold's scientific work. For example, in 2007, he was given the Award for Distinguished Professional Contributions to Applied Research by the American Psychological Association and the Lifetime Achievement Award from the Section for the Promotion of Psychotherapy Science of the Society of Counseling Psychology.

contextual factors of the psychotherapy endeavor" (p. 23). Among these "contextual factors" are the alliance, the therapist, the relationship, client expectations, the presence of a plausible rationale and set of procedures, allegiance of the therapist and client to the rationale and procedures, and so forth.

To determine which side of the debate--the medical model or the contextual model--was supported by the scientific evidence, Wampold conducted elaborate analyses and meta-analyses of decades of research on therapeutic effectiveness. *The results were clear and unambiguous: the scientific evidence showed that the contextual model is correct and the medical model is wrong. In other words, the evidence showed that it is not techniques that are responsible for therapeutic outcome but certain other factors in the therapeutic situation that are common to all therapeutic systems.*

The following is a summary of Wampold's major findings: *First, psychotherapy is highly effective.* After reviewing the meta-analyses of psychotherapy research that had been conducted since the late 1970s, Wampold (2001) concluded that psychotherapy is robustly effective. He wrote,

> From the various meta-analyses conducted over the years, the effect size related to absolute efficacy appears to fall within the range of .75 to .85. A reasonable and defensible point estimate for the efficacy of psychotherapy would be .80, a value used in this book. This effect would be classified as a large effect in the social sciences, which means that the average client receiving therapy would be better off than 79% of untreated clients.... Simply stated, *psychotherapy is remarkably efficacious.* (pp. 70-71)

This finding was neither new nor controversial. Previous reviews and meta-analyses had made it clear that psychotherapy is highly effective (e.g., Bergin & Lambert, 1978; Grissom, 1996; Lambert & Bergin, 1994; Lipsey & Wilson, 1993; Smith, & Glass, 1977; Smith et al. 1980).

Second, no therapeutic approach is any more effective than any other therapeutic approach. This finding is in line with other reviews and meta-analyses which show that no particular therapy has proven itself to be more effective than any other therapy (e.g., Bergin

& Lambert, 1978; Lambert & Barley, 2001; Lambert & Bergin, 1994; Luborsky et al., 1975; Orlinsky et al., 1994; Rachman & Wilson, 1980; Robinson, Berman, & Neimeyer, 1990; Seligman, 1995; Shapiro & Shapiro, 1982).

In specific regard to this chapter and the debate about ESTs, this finding means that so-called "empirically supported" psychotherapies such as CBT are no more effective than traditional psychotherapies. Also, when coupled with the fact that psychotherapy is highly effective, the finding means that all therapeutic approaches, including traditional psychotherapies, are effective, and equally so. In more strident moments, I have wanted to ask my colleagues on the other side of this debate, "What part of 'equal' do you not understand?" By continuing to insist that so-called "empirically supported" approaches are more effective than other approaches, they are apparently taking the position that their approaches are "more equal" than others! Wampold's research makes it clear, however, that no therapeutic approach is any more effective than any other therapeutic approach. And in regard to the question of which therapies are "empirically supported," the answer is: they are all "empirically supported" because the evidence shows that they are all effective, and equally so. Thus, in that sense traditional psychotherapies are just as "empirically supported" as CBT and other such approaches whose proponents try to exercise a monopoly on that designation.

Third, no therapeutic techniques are any more effective than any other therapeutic techniques. This finding agrees with other studies (e.g., Gloaguen, Cottraux, Cuchert, & Blackburn, 1998; Lipsey & Wilson, 1993; Shadish, Navarro, Matt, & Phillips, 2000) that show no significant differences in the effectiveness of techniques from various therapeutic approaches. To make sure his findings were correct on this point, Wampold took the additional step of analyzing the research that focused specifically on the efficacy of techniques. He found no evidence for "specificity," meaning he found no evidence to support the view that specific techniques are responsible for therapeutic outcome. As Wampold (2001) put it, "In this chapter, research designed particularly to detect the presence of specificity were (sic) reviewed. The results of studies using component designs, placebo control groups, mediating constructs, and moderating constructs consistently failed to find evidence for specificity" (pp. 147-148).

Near the end of his book Wampold (2001) reiterated this finding and admonished clinicians to have humility about their techniques. He said:

> The evidence in this book has shown that specific ingredients are not active in and of themselves. Therapists need to realize that the specific ingredients are necessary but active only in the sense that they are a component of the healing context. Slavish adherence to a theoretical protocol and maniacal promotion of a single theoretical approach are utterly in opposition to science. Therapists need to have a healthy sense of humility with regard to the techniques they use. (p. 217)

In a more recent book on evidence-based practice, Wampold (2005) contributed a chapter titled "Do Therapies Designated as ESTs for Specific Disorders Produce Outcomes Superior to Non-EST Therapies? Not a Scintilla of Evidence to Support ESTs as More Effective than Other Treatments." According to my old *Merriam-Webster Dictionary* (1965), the word "scintilla" is a noun meaning "spark" or "trace" (p. 771). Thus, Wampold was saying that there is not a "spark" or "trace" of scientific evidence to support ESTs as more effective than other treatments!

In specific regard to this chapter and the debate about ESTs, Wampold's (2005) findings mean that so-called "empirically supported" techniques are no more effective than the techniques of traditional psychotherapies. Going even further, Wampold's findings show that techniques, in and of themselves, are not responsible for therapeutic outcome. These scientific findings are a devastating blow to ESTs, which are based on the medical model assumption that specific techniques are responsible for therapeutic healing. As Wampold (2001) said, "The evidence presented in this book has undermined the scientific basis of the medical model of psychotherapy, thus destroying the foundation on which ESTs are built" (p. 214).

Fourth, therapeutic effectiveness is the result of certain factors in the therapeutic situation that are common to all therapeutic systems. Wampold (2001) referred to these as "contextual factors" and showed that these factors, rather than modalities and techniques, are responsible for client improvement and therapeutic outcome.

In specific regard to this chapter and the debate about ESTs, this finding means that the debate about which modalities and techniques are "empirically supported" is meaningless. Simply put, if contextual factors, instead of modalities and techniques, are responsible for therapeutic benefits, then it is pointless to talk about which modalities and techniques are "empirically supported" because modalities and techniques are not responsible for therapeutic outcome anyway! This finding also means that proponents of traditional psychotherapies have no scientific obligation to prove that their modalities and techniques are "empirically supported" because, again, modalities and techniques are not responsible for therapeutic outcome anyway! Instead, we should focus our scientific efforts on the factors in psychotherapy that are actually responsible for therapeutic benefits.[4]

The Place of Theory and Techniques in the Contextual Model

One might conclude from what has been said that theories and techniques have nothing to do with therapeutic outcome. In one sense, this is true because Wampold's (2001) research shows that theories and techniques, *in and of themselves*, have very little, if anything at all, to do with therapeutic benefits. On the other hand, while they have no *inherent* power to heal, theories and techniques *do* contribute to therapeutic outcome by providing a credible rationale and set of procedures that serve as a vehicle for the therapeutic work and by expressing, and serving as a conduit for, other factors in the therapeutic situation known to be responsible for outcome. In other

---

[4] Adding another devastating blow to the medical model, Miller, Wampold, and Varhely (2008) reported findings from a meta-analyses of treatment modalities for youth disorders and Benish, Imel, and Wampold (2008) reported findings from a meta-analysis of treatments for posttraumatic stress disorder (PTSD). In both studies, the results showed that no specific treatment modality was any more effective than any other treatment modality, suggesting once again that contextual factors--not specific modalities or techniques--are responsible for therapeutic outcome. The findings relative to PTSD are not only a blow to the medical model but also to cognitive-behavioral therapy (CBT) which has been viewed by many as the ideal treatment for PTSD.

words, in their role and function as contextual factors found in all therapeutic systems, theories and techniques *do* contribute to therapeutic outcome.

Thus, Wampold would support cognitive-behavioral therapists who explain to clients that their depression is due to negative thoughts and then proceed to show the client how to change those thoughts using the "specific ingredients" of CBT, meaning the specific techniques designed for thought modification. In the same way, Wampold would support psychoanalysts who tell their clients that their depression is due to unconscious conflicts and that through analytic techniques they can uncover those conflicts and alleviate their depression. However, unlike the clinicians using these approaches (probably), Wampold does not believe that the theories and techniques, in and of themselves, are responsible for alleviating the depression. Instead, he believes other factors in the therapeutic situation are responsible for the therapeutic benefits. Thus, paradoxically, one can say that theories and techniques have nothing to do with therapeutic benefits and, in the same breath, one can also say that theories and techniques *do* contribute to therapeutic benefits. The key to this apparent conundrum is to understand that while theories and techniques are not effective in and of themselves, they are effective in the sense that they provide a credible rationale and set of procedures for the therapeutic work and they serve as expressions of, and conduits for, other factors in the therapeutic situation that are known to contribute to outcome such as the alliance, the therapist, the relationship, and so forth.

Factors Responsible for Therapeutic Benefits

More than 70 years ago, Rosenzweig (1936) wrote an article titled *Some Implicit Common Factors in Diverse Methods of Psychotherapy: "At Last the Dodo Said, 'Everyone has won and all must have prizes.'"* Rosenzweig was the first to suggest that all therapies are effective due to certain factors that are common to all therapeutic approaches.[5]

---

[5] The reference to the Dodo is from *Alice in Wonderland* where the Dodo bird who, after watching a race, decided that everyone had won. The point is that every therapy "wins" or is as effective as any other therapy. Since the publication of

In 1991, Frank and Frank published *Persuasion and Healing: A Comparative Study of Psychotherapy*. In the tradition of Rosenzweig, the authors took the position that therapeutic effectiveness is due to factors common to all therapeutic systems. Wampold (2001), who based his "contextual model" on Frank and Frank's thesis and list of four major "common factors," said,

> The contextual model explains the benefits of psychotherapy by postulating that the "aim of psychotherapy is to help people feel and function better by encouraging appropriate modifications in their assumptive worlds, thereby transforming the meaning of their experiences to more favorable ones" (Frank & Frank, 1991, p. 30). The components common to all therapies include (a) an emotionally charged confiding relationship with a helping person; (b) a healing setting that involves the client's expectations that the professional helper will assist him or her; (c) a rationale, conceptual scheme, or myth that provides a plausible, although not necessarily true, explanation of the client's symptoms and how the client can overcome his or her demoralization; and (d) a ritual or procedure that requires the active participation of both client and therapist and is based on the rationale underlying the therapy. (pp. 204-205; see Wampold, 2001, pp. 24-26, for more information on the four factors).

The four factors above provide a basic framework for the contextual model. The four factors can be broken down further into more specific "common factors" such as the alliance, the therapist, the relationship, client expectations, and so forth. Taken together, these are the elusive "healing factors" in psychotherapy. It is ironic that the factors that were almost completely ignored by proponents of ESTs and the medical model have now been identified as the effective ingredients in psychotherapy! To adapt a sacred quotation, **"The stone that the builders rejected has now become the cornerstone."**

How much influence do contextual factors have on therapeutic outcome? Perhaps the best known "pie chart" for contributions to

---

Rosenweig's article in 1936, the idea that therapeutic effectiveness is due to common factors has been referred to as the "Dodo Bird Verdict."

outcome is that of Lambert (1992, p. 97) who partitioned the variability in improvement of psychotherapy clients into four parts. He attributed 40% to extratherapeutic factors, 15% to expectancy (placebo effects), 15% to techniques, and 30% to common factors. However, as Wampold (2001) pointed out, these percentages are somewhat arbitrary. Lambert (1992) did not use meta-analytic techniques to arrive at the percentages and admitted that "no statistical procedures were used to derive the percentages" and that they appeared "somewhat more precise than perhaps is warranted" (p. 98). Nevertheless, even using Lambert's questionable percentages, if one combines his expectancy or placebo effects (15%) with his common factors (30%), this means that contextual factors (expectancy plus common factors) account for 45% of the variance versus only 15% for techniques. In other words, even in Lambert's schema, contextual factors account for three times as much of the variance as techniques!

Using sophisticated meta-analytic techniques, Wampold derived percentages of variability due to specific contextual factors. Summarizing these, Wampold (2001) said,

> Placebo treatments, which contain some but not all common factors, account for 4% of the variability in outcomes…. One prominent common factor studied is the working alliance; the proportion of variability in outcomes due to this one factor is substantial (about 5%). Moreover, allegiance, another common factor, accounts for up to 10% of the variability in outcomes. Finally, the variance due to therapists within treatments accounts for somewhere between 6 and 9% of the variance in outcomes. (p. 206)

Perhaps more striking is Wampold's (2001) estimate of the variance attributable to common factors in the effects of psychotherapy. He said, "…at least 70% of the psychotherapeutic effects are general effects (i.e., effects due to common factors)." He then went on to say that specific effects, i.e., techniques, "account for at most 8 % of the variance…." (p. 207). In regard to variability of outcomes, Wampold noted that although previous work had suggested that specific ingredients are responsible for 1% of the variability, that figure failed to take into account therapist effects. Wampold's own analysis suggested that techniques, *in and of themselves*, may very well account for *none* of the variance! Wampold stated his conclusion as follows:

> Lest there be any ambiguity about the profound contrast between general and specific effects, it must be noted that the 1% of the variability in outcomes due to specific ingredients is likely a gross upper bound.... Clearly, the preponderance of the benefits of psychotherapy are due to factors incidental to the particular theoretical approach administered and dwarf the effects due to theoretically derived techniques. (p. 209)

To put it simply, techniques have little, if anything at all, to do with therapeutic outcome, whereas contextual factors have powerful effects on therapeutic outcome.

Implications

The findings summarized in this chapter not only undermine the foundations of ESTs and the medical model that created them, but they also have other important implications. These implications, along with some recommendations, are presented below.

First, humanistic-existential (HE) psychologists and other proponents of traditional psychotherapies should shift the debate about ESTs to a new battleground. The old battleground was based on the assumption that we should be able to prove the scientific validity of modalities and techniques. The "rules of engagement" called for efficacy studies under controlled conditions where a particular modality or technique was compared to another modality or technique (or to a placebo group) in an effort to prove its efficacy. The findings presented in this chapter make it clear that this old battleground is now obsolete. The scientific debate, whether some recognize it or not, has shifted to a new venue. The new venue is based on the assumption, supported by the findings summarized in this chapter, that therapeutic benefits are not due to modalities and techniques but, rather, to certain "contextual factors" common to all therapeutic systems. I would urge humanistic psychologists and other proponents of traditional psychotherapies to recognize that the debate has shifted to this new venue. If we do this, we can win the scientific debate because the evidence clearly shows that (a) all psychotherapies are effective, and equally so; (b) modalities and techniques (including ESTs) have little or nothing to do with therapeutic outcome; and (c) contextual factors, not modalities and techniques, are responsible for therapeutic effectiveness. These findings deconstruct the whole medical model notion of ESTs and provide scientific support for traditional psychotherapies.

Second, researchers and clinicians associated with HE psychology and other traditional psychotherapies should reduce efforts to prove that particular modalities and techniques are more efficacious than others and focus instead on understanding the factors that are actually responsible for therapeutic outcome. Much work needs to be done to understand contextual factors and exactly how they contribute to therapeutic effectiveness. Bohart and Tallman (Bohart & Tallamn, 1999; Tallman & Bohart, 1999) have provided an excellent example of what is needed. Their work has focused on the client as a "common factor" in therapy and as an active agent in the healing process, a perspective that challenges the medical model view that the client is the passive recipient of "treatments." Rennie's (1990, 1994, 1997) work also demonstrates how the client is active in therapy and exercises control of the therapeutic process. Once we throw off the shackles of medical model thinking and begin to focus on the factors that are actually responsible for therapeutic healing, we will radically "revision" psychotherapy. This is an exciting opportunity for researchers and clinicians who wish to make substantive contributions to our understanding of therapeutic healing.

Third, researchers and clinicians associated with HE psychology should focus increased attention on HE therapies to identify "additional benefits" these therapies may provide in addition to the alleviation of emotional problems. ESTs and "evidence-based practice," in accord with the medical model that created them, focus almost entirely on the elimination of symptoms and disorders. HE therapies, by contrast, purportedly provide clients with "additional benefits" that go beyond the alleviation of symptoms and problems. It would be relatively simple to design a research project that asks, "What, if anything, does existential psychotherapy (for example) offer clients that CBT (for example) does not?" These "additional benefits," if indeed they exist, may not be reimbursable by health insurance companies, but their identification and publication would show what HE therapies can offer clients as contrasted to the offerings of technique-dominated ESTs which appear, on the surface at least, to be quite barren. To conduct such a research project, one could generate a list of possible "additional benefits" of psychotherapy and ask clients from two therapies, e.g., existential therapy and CBT, to indicate which, if any, "additional benefits" they received from their respective therapeutic experiences. Likert-like scales could be used so clients could indicate to what degree each of these "additional benefits" was part of their therapeutic experience and to what degree they considered each benefit important. (By providing this outline, I am hoping that some graduate student will be inspired to take this on as a dissertation project!).

Fourth, training programs in clinical and counseling psychology should include a strong focus on the contextual factors so that students do not spend an undue amount of time learning modalities and techniques to the neglect of cultivating skills, attitudes, and values associated with the factors actually responsible for therapeutic effectiveness. Unfortunately, most graduate training programs focus generous amounts of time on modalities and techniques and relatively little time on helping students develop the qualities and skills associated with contextual factors. Based on the evidence presented in this chapter, programs that put all their eggs in the modality and technique basket are short-changing their students' education. Such programs, it could be said, are "majoring in minors and minoring in majors." In regard to the focus of training, the research already provides considerable guidance. For example, Orlinsky et al. (1994) reviewed more than 2,000 studies and identified several therapist-related variables that consistently have been shown to contribute to therapeutic outcome. Based on this research, Lambert and Barley (2002) published the following list:

> Therapist credibility, skill, empathic understanding, and affirmation of the patient, along with the ability to engage with the patient, to focus on the patient's problems, and to direct the patient's attention to the patient's affective experience, were highly related to successful treatment. (p. 22)

To show how important such training can be, even in regard to one therapist-related skill, one only has to look at the research by Lafferty, Beutler, and Crago (1991) who examined differences between less effective and more effective trainees. The findings showed that empathy was a differentiating variable between the two groups, i.e., less effective trainees had significantly lower levels of empathy than more effective trainees. This led the researchers to say, "The present study supports the significance of therapist empathy in effective psychotherapy. Clients of less effective therapists felt less understood by their therapists than did clients of more effective therapists" (p. 79).

Similarly, Burns and Nolen-Hoeksema (1992) examined the role of empathy in the treatment of depression by cognitive-behavioral therapists. The findings were clear: "The patients of therapists who were the warmest and the most empathic improved significantly more than the patients of the therapists with the lowest empathy ratings.... (p. 447)." As a result of this finding and wanting to be as effective as possible, the CBT clinic began asking patients to complete a form after every session indicating the level of their therapist's empathy.

The point is this: If one therapist-related variable such as empathy can have such a profound effect on therapeutic outcome, one can only wonder what the effect might be if training focused on an aggregate of therapist-related variables and other contextual factors known to contribute to therapeutic outcome. Clearly, if our goal is to turn out highly effective therapists, this is the area on which training should focus.

Fifth, training programs in clinical and counseling psychology should consider enlarging or changing the emphasis in their selection criteria. Peter Breggin (1991) described how most training programs select students. He wrote:

> Training programs for psychotherapists…are not even trying to screen their applicants to find good, kind people who will become loving and understanding therapists. They are competing with other programs for the students with the highest test scores, the best college grades, and the most impressive academic recommendations. (p. 406)

For decades those of us who have taught in graduate training programs have observed that some students, with average or lower scores on standardized tests, nevertheless turned out to be highly effective psychotherapists. Conversely, some extremely bright students, as measured by standardized tests, turned out to be average (or even worse) psychotherapists. The findings summarized in this chapter may provide a clue to this puzzle. If contextual factors (e.g., the alliance, the therapist, the relationship, etc.) are responsible for therapeutic effectiveness, an applicant's intellectual and academic abilities may not be sufficient to guarantee success as a psychotherapist. While a certain level of intellectual ability is obviously required for graduate training, it may be that personal characteristics such as caring, warmth, and empathy, along with the ability to structure a therapeutic situation and create an intimate, healing environment, are more critical to success as a therapist than are intellectual and academic abilities. Programs might get better students–and better future clinicians–if selection criteria put less emphasis on standardized test scores and more emphasis on the personal and interpersonal skills and qualities of applicants.

Sixth, when evaluating current graduate students on their clinical abilities, training programs in clinical and counseling psychology should avoid focusing on theoretical and technical knowledge to the exclusion of the personal and interpersonal qualities and abilities of the student. The evidence summarized in this chapter suggests that it would be more helpful (and scientifically more defensible) to emphasize personal and interpersonal qualities and skills related to contextual factors. For example, evaluators should ask, "Is this student able to establish an effective working alliance with clients? Does the student exhibit the personal and interpersonal qualities and skills that we know are associated with the ability to form healing relationships? Does the student extend warmth, empathy, and respect to clients? Is the student able to structure and use the therapeutic situation to promote client improvement?" It might even be worthwhile to ask, "Do the clients of this student tend to get better?" This is not to suggest that client improvement or lack of improvement should be the main criterion by which students are judged. Certainly, the kinds of clients a student works with, the level of experience and training of the student, the fact that practicum rotations can interfere with therapy and other factors outside students' control can affect therapeutic success. Nevertheless, if the clients of a student do indeed tend to get better, this suggests that the student may be doing something right (even if his or her theoretical and technical knowledge is not perfect) and this fact should receive appropriate consideration in the overall evaluation of the student.

Conclusion

Rollo May (1983) warned us about the American tendency to focus on techniques to the neglect of other, deeper dimensions of psychotherapy. As May knew, America is a frontier nation and we want practical, simple solutions, even to complex problems. Above all, we want to "fix things." It is no accident that behaviorism thrived in America and that CBT and other short-term, technique-dominated approaches are popular with American clinicians. In time, I suspect we will view psychology's current obsession with techniques and "quick fixes" as an historical expression of this cultural tendency gone wild in a time of economic fears brought on by managed care. In the meantime, we have a debate of historical proportions on our hands. I would urge HE psychologists and other proponents of traditional psychotherapies to embrace the scientific findings summarized in this chapter. We should embrace these findings not only because they undermine so-called ESTs and will help us win the current debate but also because they show that it is not modalities and techniques that heal the client but other factors in the therapeutic situation, most of which have to do with the deeply human experience of two persons reaching out to each other. One reaches out for help; the other reaches out to give it. And while some of us may have to relinquish cherished beliefs that HE approaches are more effective than other approaches, we should welcome the information that therapeutic healing, wherever it occurs, is due in large measure to such human factors as the strength of the alliance, the qualities of the therapist, and the nature of the therapeutic relationship. The research findings on contextual factors are a powerful confirmation of what HE psychologists have maintained for years: It is not theories and techniques that heal the suffering client but the human dimensions of therapy and the "meetings" that occur between therapist and client as they work together. While writing this chapter, I thought often of Carl Rogers. His prescient insights always amaze me. If he were alive today, I suspect this "new" information about what heals in psychotherapy would cause him to smile. He was the first to discover, and raise to the level of theory, that what most clients need is simply a therapist in whom healer and human are seamlessly joined, one who knows how to create a healing context and a therapeutic relationship where empathy, respect, and genuineness are offered to the client, as one might extend one's hand to a friend who has fallen.

*I would argue that humanistic psychology did not
lose its power and influence because of its
shortcomings and mistakes. We would have
survived those. Instead, humanistic psychology lost
its power and influence, in large measure, because
its liberating vision was a threat to those who were
committed to conservative ideologies. Humanistic
psychology, like the idealism of the 1960s, has
difficulty surviving in a culture where social
conservatives, fundamentalist preachers, and right-
wing fanatics hold the power.*

Chapter Five

Why Humanistic Psychology Lost Its Power and Influence
in American Psychology: A Political Analysis

*Chapter Overview: Why did humanistic psychology lose its power
and influence in American psychology? Previous answers have
focused on the historical shortcomings of the humanistic movement,
but this chapter suggests that two outside force--conservative forces
in the larger culture and mainstream American psychology--played
major roles in undermining the humanistic vision. The chapter
emphasizes that the values of humanistic psychology are incompatible
with some of the basic views of mainstream clinical psychology and
with the conservative ideologies that have increasingly gained power
in American culture since the 1960s.*

Once upon a time, for a brief and shining moment, humanistic
psychology was a dominant force in American psychology.
Humanistic psychology arose to power in the 1950s and 1960s as a
reaction, in part, to the deterministic and pathologizing nature of
Freudian psychology and the mechanistic assumptions and practices
of behaviorism. By the late 1960s, humanistic psychology had grown
into a major "third force" in American psychology (Goble, 1978). In
1968, Abraham Maslow (1954, 1962, 1966, 1971, 1976), a major
architect of the new movement, was elected president of the
American Psychological Association (APA). Carl Rogers (1942,

1951, 1959, 1970, 1972, 1977), who had earlier served as president of the APA, was widely known as the man who had developed "client-centered therapy" and was regarded by many as the most influential psychologist in the nation. Rollo May (1959, 1972, 1974, 1980, 1983, 1984), who had brought existential psychology from Europe to America and placed it under the umbrella of humanistic psychology, was viewed as one of the major existential psychologists in the world. Other luminaries associated with the early history of humanistic psychology included Gordon Allport, George Kelly, Gardner Murphy, Henry Murray, Otto Rank, Viktor Frankl, Erich Fromm, Charlotte Buhler, Virginia Satir, Thomas Szasz, Alan Watts, R. D. Laing, Kurt Lewin, Fritz Perls, Ludwig Binswanger, James Bugental, Ernest Becker, Aldous Huxley, Paul Tillich, and Martin Buber.[6]

Humanistic psychology also had a powerful impact on American culture. Millions of everyday Americans turned to psychotherapy, encounter groups, and other growth-oriented experiences. Schools, churches, colleges, and even corporations embraced humanistic ideals and offered classes designed to enhance personal growth, interpersonal relations, and organizational development. Like a powerful symphony, the humanistic movement built toward a culture-shaking crescendo that reached its peak in the early 1970s.

Today, the symphony hall is notably quieter, and the orchestra plays to a much smaller audience. Maslow, Rogers, May, and so many others in that "first generation" are now gone. Deterministic, mechanistic, and pathologizing models once again dominate clinical psychology--despite the fact that psychotherapy research clearly supports humanistic values and perspectives (see Elkins, 2007; Elliott, 2002; Wampold, 2001, 2007). Strangely, compared to its heyday in the 1960s and early 1970s, humanistic psychology has relatively little power or influence in American psychology. This is especially odd given that many humanistic ideas have infused mainstream psychology (e.g., the power of the therapeutic relationship and the focus on strengths of clients). Unfortunately, many contemporary psychologists know little about humanistic psychology and rely, instead, on negative stereotypes and

---

[6] For an excellent overview of the early history of humanistic psychology, see Aanstoos, Serlin, & Greening, 2000. For more complete histories, see DeCarvalho, 1991; Goble, 1978; Taylor, 1999b; Welch, Tate, & Richards, 1978.

misinformation. As Taylor and Martin (2001) put it, "Mainstream psychologists, if they have any name recognition at all when asked about the movement, think of humanistic psychology as unscientific, guilty of promoting the cult of narcissism, and a thing of the past" (p. 25).

The Question Addressed in This Chapter

The question addressed in this chapter is "What happened?" How did a movement as powerful and culture-changing as humanistic psychology almost disappear in only 30 years? What crushed the humanistic vision and resurrected in its place the same old mechanistic models, deterministic protocols, and pathologizing tendencies of the past? *In short, why did humanistic psychology lose its power and influence in American psychology?*

The question is important because it goes to the heart of whether or not the humanistic vision is viable. For example, if humanistic psychology was nothing more than a "grand experiment" of the 1960s that lost its power and influence because of *inherent* flaws in its values, ideals, and perspectives, then we must either do a radical revision of the movement or perhaps just cast it onto the dump heap of other experiments in the history of psychology that were fatally flawed. On the other hand, if humanistic psychology lost its power and influence because of *outside* forces that wanted to destroy it, then the humanistic vision may still be valid and viable. Indeed, humanistic values, ideals, and perspectives may be more needed in American psychology today than in the past.

The question is also important because it has implications for the future of humanistic psychology. If we lost our power and influence because of inherent weaknesses, our future strategy must include focusing on those weaknesses and doing what we can to correct them. However, if we lost our power and influence because of *outside* forces, then we must identify those forces, determine if they are still operative, and do what we can to counteract them. These two strategies are not mutually exclusive, but the answer we give to the question posed in this chapter will determine our emphasis.

Previous Answers to the Question

The question addressed in this chapter is not new. Others have raised the question and suggested various answers (e.g., Bugental & Bracke, 1992; Buss, 1979; Cain, 2003; Gendlin,1992; Girogi, 2005; Smith, 1990; O'Hara, 1996, 2001; Taylor, 1999a; Taylor & Martin, 2001; Wertz, 1998).

Cain's (2003) article is especially worthy of note because it was inspired by Old Saybrook II (see also Warmoth, 2001; Elkins, 2000) and is a comprehensive and thought-provoking contribution to the current dialogue about the future of humanistic psychology. As much as I like Cain's article, I disagree with some of his ideas and, in the spirit of dialogue, I would like to highlight these as counterpoints to my own perspective.

First, Cain (2003) gave several reasons that, in his view, humanistic psychology failed to advance. His list included paucity of natural science research, lack of publications in mainstream journals, lack of effective organization, lack of political savvy, a maverick attitude toward mainstream psychology, and having to contend with negative stereotypes. It is hard to disagree with Cain's list. Clearly, he has put his finger on some weaknesses of humanistic psychology. Nevertheless, I find his list troubling. By focusing almost exclusively on the shortcomings of humanistic psychology, he essentially "blames the victim." In fact, Cain (2003) said that a major intent of his article was "to identify how we undermine our own progress and influence" (p. 11). In regard to mainstream psychology, he suggested that we give up our maverick ways and "invest ourselves less in being adversarial and more in assuming a cooperative attitude and identifying with what is right about psychology…." (p. 19)

Our posture toward mainstream psychology is an important issue, and I suspect Cain is right that some of us could use a little "attitude adjustment." However, I have concerns about Cain's suggestion that we give up our maverick ways. It is not that I am attached to the word "maverick" (especially since it was so widely used--some might say misused--in the presidential campaign of 2008), but I believe the word points to something that we must not lose as we look to the future of the humanistic movement. "Maverick" is a ranching term that refers to a range animal (e.g., a calf, cow, or steer) that is unbranded or that refuses to be part of the herd. If humanistic psychology had truly transformed American psychology, I might agree that it is time for us to give up our maverick ways and join the herd. However, the humanistic revolution was clearly aborted and mainstream American psychology is arguably more mechanistic, reductionistic, deterministic, and anti-humanistic today than it was before the revolution started. *Thus, in contrast to Cain, I would argue that humanistic psychology should enthusiastically embrace its maverick tradition and become even more outspoken in confronting the disastrous directions of contemporary mainstream psychology.*

Second, Cain (2003) implies that the humanistic movement would have advanced if only we had been better researchers, politicians, organizers, collaborators, and so on. In other words, he believes the humanistic movement committed *suicide*. I would argue that it was *murdered*. Although we may have shot ourselves in the foot a few times, those injuries were not fatal. The real death blows--I will argue in this chapter--came from *outside* the humanistic movement.

This is not to deny the historical shortcomings of humanistic psychology. Clearly, we must analyze our mistakes and do what we can to correct them as we move into the future, and this is why Cain's article and others like it are so important. But in this chapter I want to provide a different perspective and thus a more complete picture by describing the destructive forces--in both American culture and mainstream psychology--with which humanistic psychology has had to contend. The remainder of this chapter is devoted to that theme.

Encounter Groups: A Case Study in Negative Stereotyping

Encounter groups were one of the most visible manifestations of the humanistic movement of the 1960s, and their fate provides an illuminating "case study" of how negative stereotypes and misinformation were used to undermine the movement.

Known by various names including T-groups, sensitivity training groups, personal growth groups, and interpersonal relations groups, encounter groups were pervasive in American culture during the 1960s and early 1970s. Carl Rogers (1970) called encounter groups "the most rapidly spreading social invention of the century" (p. 1). Interestingly, the encounter group movement was a grass roots phenomenon that sprang up and blossomed outside the formal academic and psychological establishments. In 1970, Rogers said:

> Most universities still look upon it with scorn. Until the last two or three years, foundations and government agencies have been unwilling to fund programs of research in this area; the established professions of clinical psychology and psychiatry have stayed aloof, while the political right wing is certain it represents a deep-seated Communist plot. I know of few other trends which have so clearly expressed the need and desire of people rather than institutions. In spite of such adverse pressures, the movement has blossomed and grown until it has permeated every part of the country and almost every kind of modern organization. (pp. 1-2)

What drew people to encounter groups? Rogers (1970) offered the following answer:

> I believe it is a hunger for something the person does not find in his work environment, in his church, certainly not in his school or college, and sadly enough, not even in modern family life. It is a hunger for relationships which are close and real; in which feelings and emotions can be spontaneously expressed without first being carefully censored or bottled up; where deep experiences--disappointments and joys--can be shared; where new ways of behaving can be risked and tried out...." (pp. 10-11)

Despite their popularity, or perhaps because of it, encounter groups generated a great deal of concern in the mainstream psychological community. In 1971, Sigmund Koch (1971) wrote an article that was highly critical of encounter groups. Koch's article, which many thought presented a distorted view of encounter groups, set off a firestorm of articles in the *Journal of Humanistic Psychology* (e.g., Apfelbaum & Apfelbaum, 1973; Arbuckle, 1973; Bennett, 1976; Dublin, 1972; Friedman, 1976; Haigh, 1971). Some of the articles seemed to generate more heat than light but others provided helpful insights into the benefits and limitations of encounter groups.

One of the criticisms leveled against encounter groups was that they often harmed participants. Smith (1975) reviewed studies on "sensitivity training" that had been reported in major publications. Because of the allegations of harm, he was especially interested in research findings related to adverse effects. Interestingly, Smith found that although a few participants experienced adverse effects as a result of their encounter group experience, the incidence was low. After reviewing the extant literature, Smith concluded, "No study yet published provides a basis for concluding that adverse effects arising from sensitivity training are any more frequent than adverse effects arising in equivalent populations not in groups" (p. 29).

In view of all this, one would think that mainstream psychology would regard encounter groups as an important historical phenomenon (at least) and as a potentially useful contemporary vehicle for helping clients and others develop greater self-awareness and more effective interpersonal skills. This, however, is not the case. In fact, if one mentions encounter groups today, the most likely response from mainstream colleagues is a rolling of the eyes and some comment about "nude marathons," "boundary violations," or that "touchy-feely stuff" from the 1960s.

Where did these negative stereotypes originate? Unfortunately, it is impossible to answer this question in a definitive way because stereotypes--like fads and trends--arise from multiple sources, most of which are impossible to trace. Nevertheless, the following information provides a partial answer to the question.

Stereotypes typically contain a little truth mixed with a lot of lies, and this is true of the stereotypes associated with the encounter group movement. For example, in regard to the "touchy-feely" stereotype, it is true that encounter groups encouraged touching and feeling. It was not unusual for group members to give one another hugs and leaders often encouraged participants to identify and express their feelings. So if it is "bad" to give hugs or to express one's feelings, then encounter groups were a hotbed of evil.

It is also true that a few "nude marathons" took place. (A nude marathon was an encounter group, typically lasting 24 to 48 hours, in which participants removed their clothing). *Time* magazine, in its February 23, 1968, edition, published an article on nude marathons being conducted in the Los Angeles area by a psychotherapist named Paul Bindrim. Although Rogers (1970) estimated that such groups comprised less than *one-tenth of one percent* of all encounter groups, nude marathons generated a great deal of media attention (for obvious reasons) and became associated with encounter groups in many people's minds.

And in regard to the stereotype about "boundary violations," it is true that a few unethical leaders took advantage of group participants. Leader abuses ranged from using questionable techniques and "exercises" to having sexual and other exploitative relationships with participants. Thus, there were abuses associated with the group movement and humanistic psychologists should never minimize the seriousness of those infractions. At the same time, it is important to remember that such incidents were rare and that the vast majority of encounter groups were positive, helpful experiences. In fact, for a grass roots movement that spanned more than a decade and involved millions of participants and thousands of leaders, it is remarkable that there were so few incidents of emotional harm. I suspect one would find more unethical therapists, damaging techniques, and incidents of harm in the history of traditional psychotherapy than in the encounter group movement.

Thus, there is little reason to believe that encounter groups were "done in" by their own faults or excesses and that they somehow "deserved" the negative stereotypes that came to be associated with the movement. *So the question remains: Where did the negative stereotypes about encounter groups originate?* To address this question, we must look at American culture and the dark clouds that were gathering as the 1960s came to a close.

In 1970, at the height of the encounter group movement, Carl Rogers warned that right-wing forces were already at work to destroy it. Rogers (1970) wrote:

> All types of intensive group experiences have come under the most virulent attack from right-wing and reactionary groups. It is, to them, a form of "brainwashing" and "thought control." It is both a Communist conspiracy and a Nazi plot. The statements made are ludicrously extreme and often contradictory. It is fair to say that it is often pictured as being one of the greatest dangers threatening our country. (p. 11)

Rogers (1970) documented several attacks from the media of his day. For example, he noted that Alan Stang, a right-wing writer, in *The Review of the News* for April, 9, 1969 asked, "Aren't our teachers being subjected to 'sensitivity training' to prepare them for the dictatorial control which is the essence of Nazism and all Socialism?" (p. 16). And in the January, 1968, issue of *American Opinion,* official organ of the John Birch Society, Gary Allen wrote an article titled: "Hate Therapy: Sensitivity Training for Planned Change." Allen alleged that sensitivity training was a left-wing conspiracy. Perhaps most ridiculous was a diatribe written by a man named Ed Dieckman, Jr., titled "Sensitivity International--Network for World Control" (as cited in Rogers, 1970, p. 11). Congressman John Rarick, a staunch segregationist, was so impressed by the piece that he read portions of it into the *Congressional Record* of January 19, 1970. The part he chose to read attacked Elizabeth D. Koontz, the first African-American president of the National Education Association, who had earlier announced a multi-faceted education program for urban children that involved Head Start and sensitivity training for parents and teachers. Koontz was accused of trying to involve the community in a "laboratory of groups exactly as in North Vietnam, Russia, and Red China" (as cited in Rogers, 1970, p. 11). It is worthy of note that a few months later this "radical" Ms. Koontz was appointed by President Nixon to be Director of the Women's Bureau of the Department of Labor.

But why were right-wing conservatives so upset about encounter groups? Rogers (1970) gave a thought-provoking answer:

> Encounter groups lead to more personal independence, fewer hidden feelings, more willingness to innovate, more opposition to institutional rigidities. Hence, if a person is fearful of change in any form, he is rightly fearful of encounter groups. They breed constructive change…. Hence, all those opposed to change will be stoutly or even violently opposed to the intensive group experience. (p. 13)

In 1977, Rogers wrote once again about the fear of change, but this time he focused on the larger American culture and the conflict that was brewing between right-wing conservatives and those committed to change and growth (whom Rogers referred to as "new persons"). Rogers (1977) said:

> Change threatens, and its possibility creates frightened, angry people. They are found in their purest essence on the extreme right, but in all of us there is some fear of process, of change. So the vocal attacks on these new persons will come from the highly conservative right, who are understandably terrified as they see their secure world dissolve, but there will be much silent opposition from the whole population. Change is painful and uncertain. Who wants it? The answer is *few*. (pp. 280-281)

Today, more than 30 years after Rogers made his sobering predictions about the increasing power of conservative forces in American culture, it is clear that he was uncannily accurate. In the last three decades we have witnessed the rise to power of Jerry Falwell, Pat Robertson, James Dobson, Rush Limbaugh, Rupert Murdoch, and a host of other right-wing conservatives who attract millions of supporters and who fill the media with narrow, and sometimes bigoted, views. Indeed, wherever one looks today, it seems that conservative forces are exerting devastating influence. The idea that there is a "vast right-wing conspiracy" in our country is no longer a joke. If there was any residual doubt, it was erased by the politics and policies of the George W. Bush administration.

Not only did *political* forces attack humanistic psychology but *religious* forces also joined the assault. For the past 30 years the Religious Right has denounced humanistic psychology as dangerous to "Biblical Christianity." Since the 1960s, conservative Christian writers have produced a spate of books condemning humanistic psychology including *Psychology As Religion: The Cult of Self-Worship* by Vitz (1977); *The Dangers of Self-Love* by Brownback (1982); *The Emperor's New Clothes: The Naked Truth About the New Psychology* by Kilpatrick (1985); *Prophets of PsychoHeresy* by Bobgan and Bobgan (1989); and *The Road to MalPsychia: Humanistic Psychology and Our Discontents* by Milton (2002). The consensus among such writers is that humanistic psychology is self-centered, narcissistic, anti-Biblical, blasphemous, counterfeit, and godless. Kilpatrick (1985) reflects the attitude of most conservative Christian writers when he says that although humanistic psychology *appears* to focus on positive things, it is actually very dangerous. Kilpatrick (1985) warned, "Humanistic psychology looks more and more like one of those seemingly benign drugs whose harmful effects do not become apparent until years later" (p. 6).

Maureen O'Hara, who worked with Carl Rogers for 18 years and more recently served as president of Saybrook Graduate School and Research Center, recalled some of her own clashes with conservative forces. O'Hara said:

> The turmoil of the late 1960s, which at times appeared as if it would result in revolution, deeply offended and scared the daylights out of the conservatives.... They believed--deeply believed--that America and the world were threatened by the ideas then in currency on the campuses and within the various social movements. The Religious Right (correctly from that point of view) identified secularism, progressive movements in general and humanistic psychology as part of that, as forces that were undermining the status quo in American life--the authority of Christian morality, patriarchy, the structure of families, white supremacy, private property, individual freedom and responsibility, and capitalism. I remember the first couple of salvos I encountered in that fight when a group of Christians picketed an AHP meeting in Indianapolis at which a "pagan" was speaking. They brought TV cameras to witness their prayers for the souls of those at the conference. I was interviewed by the TV anchor and took a moderate constructivist and "empathic" position. My words were not aired but the chanting and prayers were featured prominently. Another early encounter was the hate-mail we received against values clarification and sex education which included an official document of the John Birch Society smeared with "blood" across the page, denouncing our program as decadent and "anti-American." (M. O'Hara, personal communication, July 12, 2007)[7]

---

[7] Throughout her career O'Hara has emphasized that humanistic psychology is about emancipation and empowerment. Similar to my emphasis in this chapter, she believes we are involved in a political struggle and must therefore learn to think and act politically. I especially recommend O'Hara's (2001) article, "Emancipatory Therapeutic Practice for a New Era: A Work of Retrieval."

Arthur Bohart, a humanistic psychologist and scholar, was also active in the humanistic movement of the 1960s. In response to my question as to why humanistic psychology lost its power and influence, he made some insightful comments about American culture and mainstream psychology. Bohart wrote:

I think cultural values, both inside and outside academia, played a role. No matter how many excesses there were in the '60s (and there were many), I still look back on that time and marvel at what it tried to achieve. It tried to achieve a time of peace, of love, and of universal acceptance (for instance, I remember people taking care of their crazy brothers rather than have them hospitalized). Yet, the '60s is derided by the mainstream. It is seen as narcissistic, indulgent, and too loose. So a time which had as its ideals people relating to one another in peace and love, which valued freedom, which prized diversity, which valued rich and colorful experience (music was everywhere, as was colorful clothing, psychedelically painted vans, etc.), and which valued things of the spirit, is derided. I think that tells us a lot about the culture we live in. It is the same kind of culture where mainstream clinical psychology cannot accept the idea that a human relationship by itself can be healing. Sure, the therapeutic alliance is important, but only as a support for the real "potent" healing of interventions. I have seen many examples where the idea that the relationship can be healing is viewed as silly nonsense. In our book (Bohart & Tallman, 1999) we quote a psychiatrist who makes fun of the idea that one's "bedside manner" can heal. David Burns (1999) says in *Feeling Good* that empathy can make you feel better temporarily, but reinforces dysfunctional thinking and in the long run won't help. A psychologist from Scandinavia that I had an exchange of articles with on evidence-based practice made fun of the idea that "con amore" conversation, as he called it, could help. And a colleague said at a North American Society for Psychotherapy Research conference a few years ago that he had had an article rejected by a prominent psychology journal because, in part, one of the reviewers made fun of the idea that the relationship can be healing. What kind of culture makes fun of the idea that relationship can be healing? It is the same culture that, around 1900, chose brutal treatment of schizophrenics over moral therapy, which essentially was healing by love, and had a success rate that is better than what we have today. Who chose that brutal treatment over moral therapy? M.D.s who claimed that moral therapy wasn't "scientific" (see Robert Whitaker's *Mad in America*, 2002). I think part of the rejection of humanistic psychology is a fear of things that aren't "tough" and "hard." How often do you hear scientists use language such as "hard science," "tough-minded," "unsentimental," "ruthless, cold logic," and "no nonsense" as if they take pride in being hard and unsentimental. Humanistic psychology is too soft, too fuzzy, too warm, too right brain. It doesn't emphasize cold logic (cognitive behavior therapy), things you can observe (behavior therapy), or materials you can ingest (drugs). Look at the current love affair with biopsychology, as if we can now believe in empathy because someone found mirror neurons. And I think this is the dominant ideology of the culture too, or at least in the power sectors of the culture. And then I suspect that humanistic psychology's emphasis on freedom is threatening to those who value rigid conservative moral values. So on the one hand you have those who find it not tough enough, and on the other hand, those who view it as too loose, and it is marginalized. So I'm not sure it is anything we did as much as we are ahead of our time and it will take awhile for the culture to catch up with us. (A. Bohart, personal communication, April 24, 2007)

Is it any wonder that humanistic psychology lost its power and influence in such a culture? Humanistic psychology is inherently incompatible with right-wing ideologies that seek to impose rigid moral values and suppress civil liberties and individual freedom. Humanistic psychology is a psychology of liberation focused on change and growth, a passionate vision that all human beings have dignity and worth. Perhaps because of the unwritten taboo against discussing politics in scholarly venues, humanistic psychologists have been reluctant to explicitly acknowledge their liberal foundations.

Yet, Buss (1979) was at least partly right when he insisted that humanistic psychology and what he called "liberal ideology" have much in common. This is one reason humanistic psychology blossomed in the liberal soil of the 1960s and wilted so quickly in the ensuing years as conservative forces regained their stranglehold on the country.

Thus, I would argue that humanistic psychology did not lose its power and influence because of its shortcomings and mistakes. We would have survived those. Instead, humanistic psychology lost its power and influence, in large measure, because its liberating vision was a threat to those who were committed to conservative ideologies. Humanistic psychology, like the idealism of the 1960s, has difficulty surviving in a culture where social conservatives, fundamentalist preachers, and right-wing fanatics hold the power.

Mainstream Psychology:
How It Undermines Humanistic Psychology

The other major reason humanistic psychology lost its power and influence in American psychology has to do with mainstream psychology. Before readers decide that my paranoid tendencies have gotten the better of me, let me hastily add that I have been a member of APA for many years, and I taught in a traditional psychology program for most of my professional life. It has been my experience that mainstream colleagues are just as ethical, professional, and caring as my humanistic colleagues. Thus, what I have to say here is not intended to be a general assault on the personal integrity or motivations of mainstream psychologists.

Nevertheless, I do believe that mainstream psychology has undermined, and continues to undermine, humanistic psychology. This undermining takes three major forms: (a) perpetuating negative stereotypes about humanistic psychology; (b) failing to acknowledge the scholarly contributions of humanistic psychology; and (c) acknowledging, but then minimizing, the contributions of humanistic psychology. I will discuss each of these below.[8]

---

[8] I use the term "mainstream psychology" to refer to the "power sectors" of American psychology, i.e., to those prominent individuals, committees, boards, councils, and so forth that have the power to determine, or significantly influence, the values and directions of American psychology. While most of these power

Perpetuating Negative Stereotypes about Humanistic Psychology

Unfortunately, mainstream psychologists sometimes perpetuate negative stereotypes about the humanistic movement, thereby damaging the reputation and credibility of humanistic psychology and those associated with this orientation. Consider, for example, how Seligman and Csikszentmihalyi (2000) characterized humanistic psychology in a special issue of the *American Psychologist* dedicated to Seligman's "positive psychology." In an apparent attempt to distance positive psychology from humanistic psychology, Seligman and Csikszentmihalyi (2000) wrote:

> Unfortunately, humanistic psychology did not attract much of a cumulative empirical base, and it spawned myriad therapeutic self-help movements. In some of its incarnations, it emphasized the self and encouraged a self-centeredness that played down concerns for collective well-being. Future debate will determine whether this came about because Maslow and Rogers were ahead of their time, because these flaws were inherent in their original vision, or because of overly enthusiastic followers. However, one legacy of the humanism of the 1960s is prominently displayed in any large bookstore: The "psychology" section contains at least 10 shelves on crystal healing, aromatherapy, and reaching the inner child for every shelf of books that tries to uphold some scholarly standard. (p. 7)

This paragraph is filled with negative stereotypes about humanistic psychology. According to the authors, humanistic psychology (a) has little empirical base, (b) is self-centered, (c) is unconcerned about others, (d) may be inherently flawed or made to appear so by its followers, (e) is associated with crystals, aromatherapy, and the "inner child," and (my favorite) (f) is even responsible, apparently, for the merchandising and displays at Barnes and Noble!

---

sectors are associated with the APA, they are not necessarily synonymous with that organization.

It is noteworthy that the authors offered no documentation for their criticisms. Unfortunately, negative stereotypes about humanistic psychology have become so ingrained in mainstream American psychology that, apparently, even respected scholars can appeal to them in a major journal of the American Psychological Association without even bothering to document their allegations![9]

Fortunately, Tom Greening and Arthur Bohart, two prominent humanistic scholars, wrote a well-documented response that was published in a later issue of the *American Psychologist*. Among other rebuttal statements, Greening and Bohart (2001) countered that "neither the theory nor practice of humanistic psychology is narrowly focused on the narcissistic self or on individual fulfillment" (p. 81). They pointed out, for example, that the *Journal of Humanistic Psychology* (of which Greening was editor for 38 years) had published more than 100 articles on such topics as "the promotion of international peace and understanding, the holocaust, the reduction of violence, and the promotion of social welfare and justice for all" (p. 81). They wryly added that the journal had published "no articles at all on crystals or aromatherapy" (p. 81). In regard to Seligman and Csikszentmihalyi's claim that humanistic psychology did not "attract much of a cumulative empirical base," Greening and Bohart pointed out that Carl Rogers is often called the father of psychotherapy research and then cited recent research showing that effect sizes for humanistic therapies are as great, and sometimes greater than, those of cognitive behavioral and psychodynamic approaches. Greening and Bohart concluded by saying, "In sum, ours is a point of view that values connection, dialogue, understanding and promotion of the welfare of others" (p. 82).

Greening and Bohart could have added that Rogers was nominated for the Nobel Peace Prize in 1987, an award not typically given to narcissistic individuals or to those whose theories promote self-centeredness and that Viktor Frankl (1963, 1978, 1986) always emphasized that self-actualization can only be attained by those who,

---

[9] This is also a good example of how major psychology journals exercise considerable power in determining what is published and what is not--a point made later in this chapter. Why did the *American Psychologist*, a major journal with a well-deserved scholarly reputation, permit these authors to make such negative statements without documenting their allegations?

in self-forgetful service, dedicate their lives to a cause greater than themselves.

Failing to Acknowledge Humanistic Contributions

Mainstream psychology also undermines humanistic psychology at times by failing to acknowledge its scholarly contributions, as the following examples show: First, Seligman (2000), mentioned above, provides a contemporary example of this problem. Seligman's positive psychology is, in many ways, a reframing of humanistic psychology's long-time emphasis on the strengths and potentials of human beings. Yet, when Seligman and Csikszentmihalyi (2000) edited the special issue of the *American Psychologist* discussed above in which hundreds of references associated with this "new" approach were cited; only Viktor Frankl and Abraham Maslow made the list. *Carl Rogers, the first psychologist to reject the pathology model and to develop a scientifically supported theory of psychotherapy that focused on the positive potentials of clients, did not appear in any of the reference lists!*

Second, Heinz Kohut (1971, 1977, 1982, 1984, 1985), who created "self psychology," also failed to acknowledge the similarities between his theory and that of Carl Rogers. Kohut, an influential psychoanalyst who served as president of the American Psychoanalytic Association and vice president of the International Psychoanalytic Association, was originally trained as a classical psychoanalyst by Anna Freud. Based on his observations of transference phenomena in certain types of clients, he eventually developed self psychology, a therapeutic approach that was widely hailed as a major innovation in the psychodynamic field. Kohut's theory focused on the development of the self in the young child and how that self can be damaged. In order to restore a client's damaged self, Kohut believed that "empathic attunement" on the part of the therapist was essential. At first Kohut believed that empathic attunement was effective because it provided the analyst with better access to the client's inner material so that more accurate interpretations could be made. In time, however, Kohut came around to a view that empathy had healing capacities within itself. As Kohut (1982) put it, "I must now, unfortunately, add that empathy per se, the mere presence of empathy, has also a beneficial, in a broad sense, a therapeutic effect--both in the clinical setting and in human life in general" (p. 397).

Does any of this sound familiar? Carl Rogers's (1951, 1959, 1972) theory of psychotherapy, first formulated in the 1940s, also focused on the development of the self in the young child and made "empathic understanding" on the part of the therapist a centerpiece of therapy. *Yet, despite the obvious similarities between Kohut's theory and that of Rogers, Kohut never mentioned Rogers in any of his writings* (Tobin, 1990). If Kohut was oblivious to the similarities between his theory and that of Rogers, other scholars were not. For example, Stolorow (1976) wrote about the similarities; Kahn (1984) published an article in the *American Psychologist* comparing the two theories; and Tobin (1990, 1991) published two articles that discussed the similarities. Thus, this is another example of a prominent clinician who failed to acknowledge humanistic contributions.

Third, spirituality has been a major topic in humanistic psychology for 40 years. In his later years Maslow (1976) wrote a book about spirituality, started the transpersonal psychology movement, and helped launch *The Journal of Transpersonal Psychology*. Humanistic and transpersonal psychologists have published dozens of articles and books on spirituality. Several graduate schools associated with the humanistic movement include spirituality as part of their curriculum (e.g., Institute of Transpersonal Psychology, California Institute of Integral Studies, and Saybrook Graduate School and Research Center). In recent years mainstream psychologists have become interested in spirituality and APA has published several books on the topic (e.g., Miller, 1999; Richards & Bergin, 1997; Richards, Hardman, & Berrett, 2007; Shafranske, 1996). Yet, with the exception of Shafranske (1996), these authors give little credit to humanistic and transpersonal psychologists for their groundbreaking and continuing work in this important area.

Other examples could be given, but these are sufficient to show how humanistic contributions are sometimes ignored, even by prominent clinicians and scholars. The truth is, humanistic psychology has made major contributions to the field. The following list highlights some of those contributions:

1. The humanistic movement was largely responsible for turning America into a "therapeutic culture" and helping enlarge the field of psychology from a small guild of about 7,000 in 1950 into a profession of over 90,000 today (see Bellah et al., 1985; American Psychological Association, 2000).

2. The humanistic movement was primarily responsible for changing society's perception of psychotherapy from a "medical treatment for mental illness" into a vehicle for personal growth and a source of support and guidance during difficult times (see Bellah et al., 1985; Elkins, 2008; Maslow, 1962, 1971; O'Hara, 1996; Rogers, 1942, 1951, 1972).

3. The humanistic movement brought spirituality under the umbrella of psychology and helped make it a legitimate area of psychological study (see Elkins, 2001; Maslow, 1976; Taylor, 1999b).

4. Humanistic scholars did groundbreaking work in the area of philosophy of research, writing about the limitations of the natural science model when applied to psychological phenomena and demonstrating the importance of phenomenological and other qualitative approaches in understanding human experience (e.g., Giorgi, 1968, 1970, 1985; Maslow, 1966; Wertz, 2001).

5. The movement helped create and promote encounter groups, arguably the most effective psychoeducational tool ever invented for helping individuals to develop greater self-awareness and more effective interpersonal skills. Relatedly, the movement demonstrated the therapeutic value of group processes and laid foundations for the widespread use of therapy groups in clinical settings today (Lieberman et al, 1973; Rogers, 1970).

6. Rogers's Person-Centered Approach (PCA) has been the focus of hundreds of research studies which overwhelmingly have confirmed the effectiveness of his "necessary and sufficient" conditions of therapy (i.e., empathy, congruence, and unconditional positive regard). (see Barrett-Lennard, 1998; Rogers, 1951, 1959).

7. Recent meta-analyses of psychotherapy research have confirmed that, on the whole, humanistic therapies are as effective as CBT and psychodynamic approaches (Elliott, 2002; Elkins, 2007; Wampold, 2001).

8. By emphasizing the importance of personal and interpersonal variables in psychotherapy, humanistic psychologists anticipated contemporary meta-analytic studies that have convincingly demonstrated that therapeutic effectiveness is due primarily to contextual factors and not to modalities and techniques (see Wampold, 2001; Elkins, 2007).

9. Rollo May almost single-handedly brought existential psychology from Europe to America in the late 1950s, introducing American psychology to this important perspective (see May, Angels, & Ellenberger, 1958; Taylor, 1999b).

10. Through their writings, existential psychologists have shown the clinical relevance of existential issues such as death, meaning, isolation, loneliness, authenticity, freedom, limitation, and responsibility (e.g., May, 1972, 1983; Schneider & May, 1995; Schneider, 2008; Bugental, 1976,1981; Yalom, 1980).

11. The humanistic movement emphasized the importance of the humanities (e.g., art, poetry, music, literature, and philosophy) for understanding human experience and for healing and enriching one's inner life. (e.g., see May, 1984, 1985; Maslow, 1962, 1971, 1976; Schneider, 2004, 2007; Schneider & May, 1995; Arons, 1994; Arons & Richards, 2001; Elkins, 1998).

12. Humanistic psychologists who embrace constructivist, narrative, feminist, and postmodern approaches have demonstrated the importance of these perspectives, especially in a postmodern age when clients struggle with the "tyranny of choice" and with multiple realities and selves (see Anderson, 1990, 1998; Leitner & Epting, 2001; O'Hara, 2001; Wadlington, 2001).

13. Contemporary humanistic thought, which focuses on such postmodern themes as alternative epistemologies, the social construction of reality, and the relativity and

limitation of abstract theoretical systems, is arguably more attuned to the postmodern age than is mainstream psychology which often seems stuck in traditional perspectives that reflect modern era assumptions (see Anderson, 1990, 1998; Elkins, 1998; Krippner, 2001; O'Hara, 1997, 2001).

14. Humanistic psychology has had a significant impact on other fields such as education, social work, nursing, group therapy, interpersonal relations, and organizational development (see DeCarvalho, 1991; Goble, 1978; Maslow, 1998; Montuori & Purser, 2001; Thomas, 2001; Welch et al., 1978).

Minimizing Humanistic Contributions

Mainstream psychologists also undermine humanistic psychology at times by acknowledging, but then minimizing, its contributions. A classic example is the professor who acknowledges that humanistic psychology made contributions to psychotherapy but then summarizes (and minimizes) those contributions by saying, "Humanistic psychology showed us the importance of having a good relationship with the client." Another example is the clinical supervisor who tells trainees that Rogerian therapy is "a good place to start." Yet another example is the professor who acknowledges that existential psychology deals with important human issues but then says, "However, existential psychology is too philosophical and unscientific to be of much use to clinicians."

Minimization is very destructive. In fact, it may be even more destructive than negative stereotypes and failing to acknowledge humanistic contributions. Minimization has a deceptive quality in that it allows one to acknowledge contributions while, at the same time, leaving the impression that those contributions were not particularly important or extensive. Minimization is "damning with faint praise." It is a "back-handed compliment" that takes away more than it gives.

Humanistic Psychology and Mainstream Psychology:
The Deeper Problem

The problems discussed above are serious but I view them as symptoms of an even deeper problem, which can be stated as follows: *The basic assumptions and values of humanistic psychology are in radical conflict with the basic assumptions and values of contemporary mainstream psychology.* I will discuss two areas that shed light on the nature of this conflict: (a) philosophy of research and (b) model of psychotherapy.

Philosophy of Research

Mainstream psychology is committed to the natural science paradigm as the "gold standard" in psychological research. Indeed, the commitment is so strong that it sometimes borders on "scientism," i.e., the philosophical position that the methods of the natural sciences should be used in all investigative endeavors. It is easy to forget that human beings choose their epistemological perspectives, which are not themselves scientifically verifiable. *In other words, to say that the natural science model should be the gold standard in psychological research is not itself a scientific statement.* It is a personal belief, a philosophical position, sometimes even an ideology. Thus, it is appropriate to ask on what basis mainstream psychology has decided that the natural science model is the gold standard for psychological research. Just because the model has been effective in the study of "things" does not necessarily mean that it is the best model for the study of psychological phenomena. Amedeo Giorgi (1968, 1970, 1985, 1992, 2001, 2005), a humanistic scholar and research philosopher, has long maintained that psychology is a unique discipline that requires its own kind of science – what he has termed "human science" (see Giorgi, 1970). Giorgi (2005) believes the discipline of psychology is still in a preparadigmatic state of development, i.e., it has not yet defined its own unique domain, clarified its subject matter, or invented research methods appropriate to that subject matter.

Humanistic psychologists are not opposed to the natural science model when it is appropriate to the phenomenon being studied. However, certain types of psychological phenomena (e.g., meaning and relationships) do not easily lend themselves to investigation by this model. Thus, many humanistic psychologists believe that one's research methods should be adapted to the phenomenon being studied instead of the other way around (see Maslow, 1966, and Giorgi, 1970).

Model of Psychotherapy

As I have already discussed in other chapters, mainstream psychology is committed to the medical model, a model that imposes a medical schema on psychotherapy, uses medical language to describe therapeutic processes, and employs medical-like techniques and procedures to "cure" or ameliorate "pathology." In contrast, most humanistic psychologists view psychotherapy not as a medical procedure but, rather, as a liberating interpersonal process that helps clients to grow so that they can solve their own problems (Elkins, 2008; O'Hara, 2003). For many of us, this is not simply a matter of theoretical disagreement but also a matter of respecting the dignity and worth of clients and refusing to endorse a model that pathologizes and disempowers those who seek our services.

Thus, there is a chasm of "Grand Canyon" proportions between the basic assumptions and values of humanistic psychology and those of contemporary mainstream psychology. We cannot even agree on how to do research or describe psychotherapy! I believe this fundamental divide best explains why the two systems are so often in conflict and why some mainstream psychologists undermine humanistic perspectives. At some level they know that if humanistic psychology were to regain its power and influence, it would represent a major threat to the contemporary psychological establishment--just as it was a threat to the psychological establishment of the 1950s and 1960s.

Implications

Perhaps the most important implication of the analysis presented in this chapter is that humanistic psychologists must think and act *politically* in order to advance humanistic psychology. *Simply put, if political forces marginalized us, then we must think and act politically in order to counteract those forces.*

What kind of action is needed? I would offer two suggestions. First, I believe we should create a "think tank" composed of a small group of our most talented and *politically astute* leaders who agree to meet on a regular basis for the sole purpose of developing strategies and tactics designed to counteract the destructive forces--in both American culture and mainstream psychology--with which humanistic psychology has to contend.

Second, I believe we should enthusiastically embrace our revolutionary tradition and launch a coordinated campaign to highlight the limitations and failures of mainstream American psychology and to describe humanistic and other progressive alternatives. For example, if we were to "flood the market" over the next few years with strategically planned books, articles, presentations, radio programs, television interviews, magazine articles, internet blogs, and other forms of communication dedicated to this theme, I believe we would (at least) provoke a much needed debate about the current state of American psychology, and we might even bring about important changes in our field.

Perhaps the greatest danger the humanistic movement faces at this point in its history is that members of the second and third generations of humanistic psychologists will abandon the radical nature of the humanistic vision. Humanistic psychology is a revolutionary perspective. Rooted in the dynamic humanism that inspired ancient Greece and that ignited the European Renaissance, humanistic psychology has the power to transform individuals, families, groups, organizations, and even cultures. It offers therapeutic and educational experiences that empower and emancipate, setting clients and students on life-long journeys of self-realization and inspiring them to take action in the world, as Rollo May (1983) might have put it. Humanistic psychology offers something that no other psychology offers: an explicit vision of what it means to be fully human and to create a life of passion and depth.

So if we truly believe that mainstream American psychology is headed in the wrong direction and that humanistic psychology can offer progressive alternatives, then we have a responsibility--perhaps even a moral obligation--to do something about it. And I know of no other group that is better qualified--by history, training, and experience--to do this than humanistic psychologists. To adapt and paraphrase Hillel: If not we, then who?

Just as the artist works with that which is "trying to become" in the painting, sculpture, poem, or novel, so the creative therapist works with that which is trying to emerge in the actualizing process of the client. The client and therapist meet in the therapeutic arena and give birth to that which is struggling to be born in the client's soul.

Chapter Six

The Deep Poetic Soul:
An Alternative Vision of Psychotherapy

Chapter Overview: The chapter is based on my Division 32 presidential address delivered in 1999 at the annual meeting of the American Psychological Association when I was president of Division 32, Society for Humanistic Psychology. Using the language of art and creativity, the chapter describes psychotherapy as an artistic endeavor that supports the client's creative becoming. Four major themes of this alternative vision are explored: (a) the "more," (b) the phenomenological experience of the emergence of the new, (c) the duende, and (d) destiny. The chapter retains the oral character of the original presentation.

This will be a different kind of presidential address. I have decided to speak both personally and poetically in the hope of communicating at the level of the heart as well as the head. I wish to speak personally because I believe all knowledge is grounded in the personal and that ultimately the best I have to give is that which I am and which I have learned in my own bones. Also, I believe that the personal, if plumbed deeply enough, has a strange way of touching the universal. So I hope as I tell my story, you will hear echoes of your own journey and feel the presence of the universal hovering nearby.

I wish to speak poetically because poetry, like all the arts, opens up dimensions of the inner life that cannot be reached in any other way. I am aware, of course, that this is an APA convention where that which is "scientific" and "scholarly" is most valued, but I am comforted by the fact that this is Division 32 where the personal and the poetic have always been not only welcomed but embraced.

My Personal Story

I grew up in the foothills of the Ozark Mountains of Arkansas. My mom had an eighth grade education and my dad worked two jobs to keep food on the table and a roof over our heads. This remote section of the country is deep in the Bible Belt and practically everyone I knew was religious. My family went to church at least three times a week, sometimes more. As a boy, I was deeply moved by the rituals of my church and by the sense of what I would now call a numinous presence.

At an early age I decided I wanted to become a minister. After graduating from high school in 1962, I attended a church-related college near Little Rock, Arkansas, to major in religion and in 1966 I became a minister. At the time I fully intended to spend the rest of my life in that profession. Today, I am no longer a minister. In fact, I am not involved with organized religion at all.

My Southern church was conservative and held fundamentalist views. It insisted that it alone had the truth and that other people, including Baptists, Methodists, Presbyterians, and especially Catholics, were all going to hell. My church had somehow managed to get a monopoly on all religious truth and everyone else was simply up the creek without a paddle. All this seems a little silly now, but that is what I was taught and what I believed as a child and young man.

Sara and I were married while I was a ministerial student. After graduation, we moved to Michigan where I became the minister of a church composed primarily of transplanted Southerners who had gone north to work in the automobile factories. To prepare my weekly sermons I often went to the university library to read books on religion and philosophy. I noticed that various religious authors kept talking about "Christian fundamentalists"--and they didn't seem to have a very high opinion of them. Even though I had a theological education of sorts, I didn't know what the word *fundamentalist* meant. As a good friend told me recently, "That's because you *was* one!" Then one day I read a book that defined fundamentalism and I was shocked to discover that I "was one!" This new meta-perspective made a small crack in my fundamentalist shell. I didn't like some of the narrow attitudes that I began to see in myself. Nourished by new thoughts and understandings, I began to grow--and that's a big mistake for a minister in a fundamentalist church.

It wasn't long until my church leaders became suspicious. They called me into a meeting and asked me a series of doctrinal questions. When I failed to give them the answers they wanted, they fired me and then a few days later they excommunicated me. So in 1968 at the ripe old age of 23 my ministerial career, barely out of the starting gates, came to a screeching halt! I spent the next two or three years trying to figure out what I was going to do with my life. In the meantime my family and I moved from Michigan to Connecticut.

In 1971 I enrolled in the Masters program in psychology at the University of Bridgeport, Connecticut. I had decided to become a counselor. I had taken nine units in my master's program before I sensed something was wrong. I went to my chairperson and asked, "When do we get to the courses that teach you how to work with people?" He said, "Dave, this is an experimental psychology program. We don't teach you how to work with people. If you want to do that, you will have to transfer to the Counseling Department in the College of Education." So you can see how naive I was about psychology.

So I transferred to the Counseling Department and that's when things became exciting. My first class was with a professor who had just returned from a workshop with Fritz Perls at Esalen Institute in California. She told us about this approach called Gestalt Therapy that seemed to be sweeping the country. I had never heard of Gestalt Therapy and I had no idea who Fritz Perls was. But when I saw his picture, I liked his white beard, long robe, and the beads he wore around his neck. He looked like an Eastern guru instead of one of those uptight-looking psychologists in my textbooks. They all reminded me of fundamentalist preachers, but Dr. Perls raised the intriguing possibility that I might someday become a psychologist guru! For some reason, perhaps because I was a child of the 60s, I found that quite appealing.

In our next class this professor introduced us to a man named Carl Rogers. She said Dr. Rogers was one of the most influential psychologists of our time and that he had developed an approach called client-centered therapy. She played an audiotape of Dr. Rogers counseling a teenage girl. I noticed that he seemed to listen well and was very kind. But toward the end of the tape I became quite irritated with this Dr. Rogers. I kept waiting for him to tell this young woman, who was obviously in need of expert advice, how to solve her problem--but he never did. I decided that if I ever became a therapist I'd surely do a better job than this Dr. Rogers in telling people what to do!

But Rogers got to me. His very human theory that emphasized empathy, congruence, and respect for the client made a lot of sense to me. I wanted to know more about this man. So I began to read his books. I was impressed by the way he wrote. It was as though he were simply talking to you, unlike most authors who seemed to delight in being as obscure as possible. Rogers touched my heart and told me what I already knew at some deep, intuitive level. Sometimes I felt he had found my diary and was telling me my own story. And when I saw the "Gloria" films, I was very touched when he told her, "Well, you look like you'd make a pretty nice daughter." Until then, I thought you had to be distant and aloof with clients. I didn't know you could talk with them like they were human beings.

Well, to make a long story short, I was home. I was a late bloomer in the humanistic movement, but I felt powerfully drawn to this approach. Until 1971 I had never heard of Fritz Perls or Carl Rogers or Abraham Maslow or Viktor Frankl or Sidney Jourard or Rollo May--but I met them all in my classes in Connecticut.

When I started thinking about doctoral programs, I heard that a man named Mike Arons at some college in Georgia had put together a list of university programs that had a humanistic emphasis. (The psychology department at the State University of Georgia in Carollton is still doing that). So I sent for the brochure and decided to apply to a humanistic school called United States International University. I chose it for three reasons: (a) It was in California, (b) Viktor Frankl was on the faculty, and (c) Esalen Institute was somewhere out there and I had heard that people went naked in the natural hot baths. Now I wasn't sure I'd ever work up the courage to do that, but as a young minister shedding his clerical collar, I definitely wanted to be geographically close to the temptation!

So in the summer of 1973 Sara and I loaded up our station wagon and, along with our two kids, we moved to San Diego. I began my doctoral program in the fall of 1973. I did get to study with Viktor Frankl and I also met Rollo May when he came to give a presentation. I worked for two years as a therapist-in-training with Dr. Everett Shostrom who had produced the Gloria films. (Dr. Shostrom is also the one who gave Division 32 the little silver oil can that has been passed from president to president since the 1970s. He said it was to be used to "oil the wheels of APA").

In 1976, near the end of my doctoral program, something happened that changed my life. I began to feel depressed and when I couldn't pull myself out of this unhappy state, I decided to enter therapy. My therapist was 73 years old and had been originally trained as a philosopher in Germany. He later became a Jungian analyst and his studies had included time at the C. G. Jung Institute in Zurich. I'll never forget my first therapy session with this old gentleman. I was nervous and had rehearsed everything I wanted to say. I got through it all but he heard the truth anyway. Near the end of the session, when I finally let him in, he said gently, "You are spiritually hungry." I started to cry. He had sifted through my long, rambling story and gone right to the heart of my problem. And he was exactly right. I *was* spiritually hungry. Organized religion no longer spoke to my soul, but I was still in need of spiritual nourishment. And for the next two years this wise, kind man was my spiritual mentor. He taught me about life and the care and feeding of the human soul.

In time my depression lifted and I felt healthy and whole. But far more important than the alleviation of my depression was the fact that my life began to change in dramatic ways. Life took on depth and passion. I experienced things more intensely. I was more in touch with my body, my passion, my creativity. I felt as though I were finally coming home to myself. I began to feel more confidence and personal power. My life, which had seemed like a television program playing in black and white, switched to living color. That therapy was the major turning point of my life, and it has influenced everything I am and everything I've done since.

My analyst died three years after my therapy ended. A few years ago I was thinking about what he had meant to my life and I wrote a poem for him, which was published in the *Journal of Humanistic Psychology* (1997). The poem is titled *My Old Jungian Analyst*. It points to an alternative vision of psychotherapy.

My old Jungian analyst would roll over in his grave
If he knew the state of psychotherapy today
Twenty years ago I walked into his office
A wounded young man
Too proud to admit the darkness
Overwhelming me
That old man would never have survived in HMOs
Would have been a failure if put to short-term test
He followed my own labyrinthine path
Got lost in the darkness with me
Sometimes had nothing to offer but his own faith
That had taken him 73 years to build
No treatment plan, no manualized procedures
His only diagnosis, "Hungry soul"
But some deep listening
That heard the distant lapping of water
The cry of whippoorwills in the dark
The murmurs of a long lost heart
And gentle words, like splints and bandages
That hold the brokenness together
While the bone mends, grows strong
And the night somehow turns to dawn
How can you measure a Rumi poem
Or calculate the beauty of a Van Gogh
Put ruler to the deepening of a heart
Or caliper to the opening of a soul
That therapy when I was a lost young man
Has touched everything I've done
How can I possibly talk of numbers
While trying to thank someone
For giving me my life (p. 41)

An Alternative Vision of Psychotherapy

Now I would like to make my alternative vision of psychotherapy more explicit. This is my personal vision and it is incomplete. Nevertheless, I would like to discuss four themes that have been important in my own thinking about psychotherapy.

Let me begin this section by saying that I am deeply concerned about the direction of psychotherapy today. I believe "managed care" and the mentality that goes with it may be the worst thing that has happened to psychotherapy in its history. This is not simply because managed care has been financially hurtful or even disastrous for thousands of good, dedicated clinicians--which it has been. *But the most damaging thing about managed care is that economic forces are redefining psychotherapy so that it will fit the "quick-fix" medical and mechanistic models demanded by a system whose ultimate concern is the bottom line.* I fear that clinical training programs, internships, and research centers will focus on the most efficient ways to alleviate psychological symptoms and that these "quick-fix" procedures will become the new definition of psychotherapy.

If this happens, something very important will be lost. I believe the most valuable thing about psychotherapy is not its ability to alleviate psychological "symptoms," as important as that is. There is "something more" that occurs in good therapy that goes far beyond symptom alleviation. I experienced this "something more" in my therapy with my old Jungian analyst. Many of you, I am sure, have experienced it in your own therapy. Also, I'm sure thousands of clients have experienced it in their therapy with you. I would even suggest that this "something more" is at the heart of what good therapy is all about.

It is not easy to define or describe this "something more." Yet, we must find ways to talk about it because it is what will be lost if we allow psychotherapy to be redefined by managed care and by those who support medical and mechanistic models of psychotherapy.

I believe the best way to talk about this "something more" is to use the language of art and creativity. In contrast to medical and mechanistic language, the language of art and creativity is rich, nuanced, and capable of describing deeper and more complex therapeutic processes. The language of art and creativity can illumine the "something more" or what I will call the "vital but almost ineffable" dimensions of psychotherapy. So in the remainder of this presentation, I want to talk about the "vital but almost ineffable" dimensions of therapy. In order to do this, I will give you a term or a phrase and then discuss what it points to.

The More

The first term is "the more" and it goes straight to the heart of the difficulty of trying to describe that which is "vital but almost ineffable" in psychotherapy. In *The Varieties of Religious Experience*, William James (1982) used the term "the more" to refer to that which lies beyond the seen world, beyond that which we can take in through our five senses. My professor Viktor Frankl used this term in class to refer to that which can hardly be said or defined, that which cannot be captured by our usual operational definitions. Rumi (1993), the Sufi mystic, put it this way: "The world of the soul follows things rejected and almost forgotten" (p. 36).

Our culture and our profession give primacy to hard facts, operational definitions, and linear ways of knowing. But these approaches often leave out "the more"--the rich, ineffable nuances and meanings that hover around the hard facts and between the lines. Denotative and linear ways of knowing tend to be narrow, constrictive, reductionistic. By contrast, connotative and nonlinear ways of knowing--metaphors, similes, images, and symbols--take us into the regions of "the more" where we often find the real substance and depth of life.

Paul Tillich (1987), speaking of the power of symbols, wrote:

All arts create symbols for a level of reality which cannot be reached in any other way. A picture and a poem reveal elements of reality which cannot be approached scientifically. In the creative work of art we encounter reality in a dimension which is closed for us without such works. (The symbol)... also unlocks dimensions and elements of our soul which correspond to the dimensions and elements of reality. A great play gives us not only a new vision of the human scene, but it opens up hidden depths of our own being. (p. 42)

Let me give you an example of "the more." A few years ago one of my graduate students spent her summer vacation living with a family in southern France. She told our class how the family prepared the evening meal. Each morning, fresh vegetables and meats were purchased at the local market and carefully washed and prepared. In the afternoon, each dish was slowly simmered on the stove and the smell of herbs and spices filled the house. In the evening, the meal was served in courses over a period of three hours or more along with several bottles of wine. The family and guests sat around the table telling stories, discussing politics, and sharing their lives with one another. When my student returned to the United States with its fast foods and prepackaged meals, she said it was the evening meals in southern France that she missed most. In America eating often tends to be just another linear event, to be done as quickly and efficiently as possible. But in southern France people seem to appreciate "the more" of dining.

What was so special to my student about those evening meals? It is not easy to put into words. It seems to have involved many different things: earthiness, soulfulness, sensuousness of sights and smells and tastes, communication, sharing, and a spirit of community. Yet all these words only point toward that ineffable "more" that my student experienced. If we were insensitive to this student's experience, we might say, "Hey! Eating is eating and as long as we take in healthy food, why would anyone want to take all day to prepare it and then spend three hours eating it?" And if we were really crass, we might make fun of the student for getting so caught up in this experience which she can't even really define, describe, or explain. I can almost hear someone saying, "Well, that's nice, dear. It sounds like you met some friendly people and had some very nice food. Now let's get on with what's really important." *It is so easy to dispense with that which is ineffable!*

Is there a metaphor here for two types of psychotherapy: one that is linear, efficient, easily defined and another that is more mysterious, circled about with awe, an experience in soul, one that touches the heart, nourishes the soul, and makes both client and therapist more human as it "follows things rejected and almost forgotten?" I think so. Albert Einstein once wrote on a blackboard: "Not everything that counts can be counted, and not everything that can be counted counts." That's important to remember when we are talking about the "vital but almost ineffable" dimensions of good psychotherapy.

The Phenomenological Experience of the Emergence of the New

The second theme is: *The phenomenological experience of the emergence of the new*. A few years ago Mark Stern invited me to participate in a symposium and talk about the "phenomenological experience of the emergence of the new" in psychotherapy. At first I had no idea what he was talking about--and Mark never told me what he meant. But the more I thought about this phrase, the more I came to believe that it pointed to something that was "vital but almost ineffable" in psychotherapy. To me, it refers to that experience in which the client begins to feel the flow of her own creative becoming. She begins to sense that she is moving toward a new but not yet definable way of being in the world.

This is not all that mysterious to those who are attuned to personal growth. When I was preparing for Mark's symposium, I contacted several friends who are among the most growthful people I know. Every one of them, without exception, understood what I meant when I asked them to describe their experience of the emergence of the new in their lives. Interestingly, they all spoke in metaphors. One woman said, "For me it's like being in a dark hallway and the door behind me has slammed shut. I know I can't go back but the door in front of me has not yet opened. I often feel panic." Another said, "I begin to realize that the old structures of my life are not working and yet I don't know what the new structures will be. They are not yet clear." Another woman said, "Once when a major change occurred in my life, I told my sister six months before it happened that I felt as though something was moving inside me, that I was in the stream and heading for a major change in my life. At the time there was no obvious reason for me to feel that way, but I knew inside that something was moving ahead."

Isabel Allende, who has written several novels that have received international acclaim, was once asked to describe how she writes. Her answer, even though she was describing creative writing, is one of the best descriptions of psychotherapy I know. Allende (as cited in Epel, 1993) said:

I write in a very organic way. Books don't happen in my mind; they happen in my belly. It's like a long elephant pregnancy that can last two years. And then, when I'm ready to give birth, I sit down. I wait for January 8th, which is my special date, and then, that day, I begin the book that has been growing inside me.

Often when I sit that day and turn on my computer or my typewriter and write the first sentence, I don't know what I'm going to write about because it has not yet made the trip from the belly to the mind. It is somewhere hidden in a very somber and secret place where I don't have any access yet. It is something that I've been feeling but which has no shape, no name, no tone, no voice. So I write the first sentence–which usually is the first sentence of the book that is the only thing that really stays. Then the story starts unfolding itself, slowly, in a long process. By the time I've finished the first draft I know what the book is about. But not before.

Somehow inside me--I can say this after having written five books--I know that I know where I am going. I know that I know the end of the book even though I don't know it. It's so difficult to explain. It is as if I have this terrible confidence that something that is beyond myself knows why I'm writing this book. And what the end of the book will be. And how the book will develop. But if you ask me what the book is about or where I am going I can't tell you. I can't tell anybody. I can't even tell myself. But I have a certainty that I would not have started the book without knowing why I'm writing it. (p. 8)

Allende has put into words a process that stands at the center of creative art and that also describes the creative nature of good psychotherapy. As many clinicians know, in good psychotherapy there is a creative process that begins to take on a life of its own as it carries the client toward some unknown yet deeply sensed destination. The client begins to experience the subtle flow of his or her own creative becoming. Like Allende, the client knows that she knows where she is going. But also like Allende, if you ask her where she is going, she can't tell you. She can't tell anybody. She can't even tell herself. But she has a certainty that she would not have started the therapeutic journey without knowing why she was making it.

From an artistic and creative perspective, therapy is the facilitation of a natural, creative process of becoming. It is an intensive endeavor in which both client and therapist focus on that which is trying to emerge or be born in the client. There is much waiting. There is not much knowing. Yet there is a strong sense that this becoming is important, perhaps even a matter of life and death. The client knows that destruction will be associated with this process. Old ways of being, old patterns, unworkable structures and relationships may have to be relinquished. She knows that before the process is over she may have to go through more anxiety, depression, and pain. Yet there is a deep, underlying faith in the process, an unshakeable sense that she is being carried by forces greater than self toward a new and ultimately more fulfilling way of being in the world.

In the book *Existence*, Rollo May (1958) said that the word *existence* comes from the root *ex-sistere* and means "to stand out" or "emerge." He said that existential psychologists see "the human being not as a collection of static substances or mechanisms or patterns but rather as emerging and becoming, that is to say, as existing" (p.12). May would have agreed with Allende. He saw psychotherapy as a creative process in which the therapist facilitates that which is "emerging" or "becoming" in the client. Just as the artist works with that which is "trying to become" in the painting, sculpture, poem, or novel so the creative therapist works with that which is trying to emerge in the actualizing process of the client. The client and therapist meet in the therapeutic arena and give birth to that which is struggling to be born in the client's soul.

I take seriously the idea that human beings go through periods of growth or becoming in which they leave old patterns behind and are carried forward toward the deeply sensed but inarticulable new. I also take seriously the idea that anxiety, depression, and other painful psychological experiences are, more often than not, signals that we have ceased to grow, that we are dying inside, suffocating in the old, untenable structures that no longer serve us in life.

Psychotherapy that focuses on "the phenomenological experience of the emergence of the new" stands at the opposite end of the continuum from the shallow, mechanistic approaches that now dominate the field. It is a deeper, more mature therapy because it relies on a deeper, more complex understanding of the human being. It honors and draws upon the vast cache of wisdom found in the world's literature, poetry, arts, philosophies, religions, and ancient healing methods. Yet, there is nothing in this deeper approach that closes its door to science or to new knowledge about the healing process.

In contrast, the technician-driven model tends to ignore this vast human context. It pays little attention, if any, to the existential and spiritual questions that may lie at the heart of the client's problems. Like the well-trained mechanic who can tune our car but has nothing to offer if we ask how to develop a better life, so the technician-therapist can remove symptoms or change behavior but knows little or nothing about nurturing the soul or helping the client to develop a deeper, more passionate existence.

I have worked in hospital, community mental health, and private practice settings. I have found that although clients often initiate therapy because of a painful emotional problem, they quickly begin to discuss their lives--the vast context and fabric of who they are, where they are going, and what is present and missing in their lives. Once clients enter this deeper process, it is almost impossible to get them to do what they consider to be "gimmicky" techniques or homework assignments directed only at symptom alleviation. They sense that they have embarked on a journey that will not only alleviate their symptoms but will also lead to a deeper, more meaningful life. In a market-driven profession that demands linear treatment plans after one or two sessions with clearly defined goals, specific methods to reach those goals, and a list of criteria for determining when therapy will be finished, the therapist who wishes to honor the deeper, creative process in clients is at a woeful disadvantage. Just as our technological society seems to have little respect for art and artists, so in psychology we do not honor the artistic therapist. Instead, the "ideal therapist" is fast becoming a left-brained, scientistic, hyper-rational technician who knows little or nothing about the existential and spiritual dimensions of life. The health care industry, driven by economics and a "quick fix" mentality, supports and rewards this kind of therapist. The faster a therapist can "get the job done" and return the suffering client to the assembly line or the corporate ladder, the more money the managed care company makes. Sadly, in America money is more important than clients' souls and therapy is becoming a "quick fix" center owned by Wall Street.

Rollo May once told a friend of mine who was immersed in the hard sciences at the time, "You need to read less science and more poetry." That says it for me. In our therapist training programs and in our profession generally, we need to read less science and more poetry. Psychotherapy is more than science and mechanistic techniques. It is also poetry and art. And it is the artistic, creative, and poetic dimensions of therapy that are most important, because they honor "the phenomenological experience of the emergence of the new." They reflect and facilitate the creative process of growing, becoming, and birthing the client's soul.

The Duende

Now, I'm going to talk about something that is truly mysterious. The term is "the duende." *Duende* is a Spanish word that originally referred to little mythical creatures or spirits that lived in the mountains in Spanish mythology. But the Spanish poet Federico Garcia Lorca used the term to refer to that mysterious energy that infuses the creative process and artistic performances. I believe this term gives us a way to describe something that is "vital but almost ineffable" that sometimes occurs in good therapy.

In his *Havana Lectures,* Federico Garcia Lorca (1992) had this to say about the duende:

Everything that has black tones has duende. And there is no truth greater. These black tones are mystery itself whose roots are held fast in the mulch we all know and ignore, but whence we arrive at all that is substantial in art. Black tones...are "a mysterious power which everyone feels but which no philosopher can explain." So then, the duende is a power and not a method, a struggle and not a thought. I have heard an old guitar teacher say that "the duende is not in the singer's throat, the duende rises inside from the very soles of one's feet."

That is to say, it is not a question of ability or aptitude but a matter of possessing an authentic living style; that is to say of blood, of culture most ancient, of creation in art. This "mysterious power which everyone feels and no philosopher can explain" is in short, the spirit of the earth. The true struggle is the duende.

The arrival of the duende always presupposes a radical transformation on every plane. It produces a feeling of totally unedited freshness. It bears the quality of a newly created rose, of a miracle that produces an almost religious enthusiasm.

All art is capable of duende. But the place that it naturally occurs is in music, dance, or spoken poetry because they require a living body for interpretation and because they are forms that perpetually live and die, their contours are raised upon an exact presence. (p. 165)

As Lorca indicates, artists know this mysterious power as the source of their creativity. One of my students, a Black woman, grew up in a family of jazz musicians. When she read Abraham Maslow's description of "peak experiences" and the realm of "Being," she was convinced that jazz musicians often tap into this dimension when they "jam" together. For a class project, she interviewed several world class jazz musicians to ask them about this. Every one of them, without exception, knew immediately what she was talking about. Using their own words, they described those special moments when an entire band is caught up in the universal. They become one with the music they are creating; there is an intense sense of flow and connection. Each player knows intuitively what the others are going to do before they do it. In those moments they become servants to the creative process, instruments through which the duende creates the new.

You may recall that Rudolph Otto (1961) in *The Idea of the Holy* talked about the "energy of the numen" (p. 5) which is present in intense encounters with the sacred. He said that this mysterious energy expresses itself as "vitality, passion, emotional temper, will, force, movement, excitement, activity, impetus" (p. 6). He said that it was "a force that knows not stint nor stay, which is urgent, active, compelling, and alive" (pp. 23-24).

Also, Mircea Eliade (1961), who served as chair of the Department of the History of Religions at the University of Chicago for seventeen years, said in his book *The Sacred and the Profane*:

The sacred is equivalent to a power, and, in the last analysis, to reality. The sacred is saturated with being. Sacred power means reality and at the same time enduringness and efficacity. The polarity sacred-profane is often expressed as an opposition between real and unreal or pseudoreal... thus it is easy to understand that religious men deeply desire to be, to participate in reality, to be saturated with power. (pp. 12-13)

When the sociologist Durkheim (1915) studied primitive cultures, he discovered a special power called "mana" that was associated with the sacred domain. When a tribesman went away to commune with the sacred, he would return to the village filled with this mysterious power. This led Durkheim to say, "The believer who has communicated with his god is...stronger. He feels within him more force, either to endure the trials of existence, or to conquer them" (p. 416).

Francine, one of my doctoral students, was born on a small island in the South Seas. For the first eight years of her life she lived in a hut with a dirt floor, spoke the language of her people, and participated in the beliefs, rituals, and daily activities of her village. One day in my humanistic-existential class I was struggling to describe this "vital but almost ineffable" idea of being filled with passion and power. Francine kept nodding her head and seemed to understand exactly what I was trying to say. She said, "That's what my people call *pakaramdam.*" Never having heard the word, I asked her to say it again. She spelled it and then pronounced it slowly – "pahk-ah-rahm-dahm." She said, "In my village when people spoke from down here (pointing to her solar plexus), it was said that they were speaking with pakaramdam. This meant that they were speaking with deep emotion, power, and passion--very different from ordinary speech."

Even as a professor, I know this force. On some days my lectures lack life. My notes lie there dead in front of me and no matter how hard I try to breathe life into them, nothing happens. My students feel the deadness and dutifully take their notes. Then on other days the duende breaks in. A deep, authentic force wells up and my words seem to flow of their own accord. The students come alive. Pakaramdam fills the classroom, and we talk from our hearts with power and passion. These are the special moments in education, perhaps the only times when real learning occurs.

What does this have to do with psychotherapy? I would suggest that duende is one name for the energy that drives the therapeutic process. It is that energy that breaks into a therapy room and transforms a client, a family, or a group that has been stuck in deadness. In their famous dialogue Carl Rogers (1989) talked about this with existential theologian Paul Tillich. Rogers told Tillich that sometimes in therapy, "I feel as though I am somehow in tune with the forces of the universe or that forces are operating through me in regard to this helping relationship" (p. 74). I would say that Rogers was experiencing the duende, that "mysterious power that everyone feels but no philosopher can explain."

This is the energy that opens up a client's heart and infuses them with new passion and power. I felt this in my therapy with Dr. Welch 30 years ago. In my group therapy work, I have seen the duende flow into a cold, defended group, break down defenses, and create a passionate community all in one evening. What is this "mysterious power that everyone feels but no philosopher can explain"? I believe it is the mystery of life itself, the powerful energies of the sacred. When we touch this domain, we are filled with the cosmic force of life itself. In these experiences we sink our roots deep into the black soil and draw power and being up into ourselves. We know the "energy of the numen" and are "saturated with power and being." We feel more rooted, grounded, centered, more in touch with the ancient and eternal rhythms of life. Power and passion well up like an artesian spring and creativity dances in celebration of life. Federico Garcia Lorca was right. The true struggle--and perhaps the only one that really matters--is with the duende.

Destiny

The final term in my alternative vision is "destiny." I believe psychotherapy is an arena for existential exploration, a place to ask, "Who am I *really*?" It is an opportunity to search for one's place in the world.

I am not sure how seriously most of us take this idea of personal destiny or authentic commitment to the "true self." But I have been impressed by the number and caliber of people who have come to the conclusion that this is what life is all about. For example, Soren Kierkegaard (1941), the founder of existentialism, believed that the goal of life is "to be that self one truly is" (p. 29). Kierkegaard (as cited in Kaufmann, 1956) said that he wanted his epitaph simply to read, "That individual" (p. 99).

Nietzsche, one of the most brilliant thinkers of all time, also believed that the task of life is to become oneself. He asked (as cited in Kaufmann, 1950), "What does your conscience say? You shall become who you are." (pp. 133-34) And in a very moving passage Nietzsche (as cited in May, 1983) wrote:

> The soul in its essence will say to herself: no one can build the bridge on which you in particular will have to cross the river of life--no one but yourself. Of course there are countless paths and bridges and demigods ready to carry you over the river, but only at the price of your own self. In all the world, there is one specific way that no one but you can take. Whither does it lead? Do not ask, but walk it. As soon as one says, "I want to remain myself," he discovers that it is a frightful resolve. Now he must descend to the depths of his existence. (p. 80)

Paul Tillich (1952), one of the most profound theologians of the twentieth century, said, "Man's being... is not only given to him but also demanded of him.... He is asked to make of himself what he is supposed to become, to fulfill his destiny." (pp. 51-52)

In his book *The Soul's Code* Jungian scholar James Hillman (1996) takes the position that each of us, like an acorn, contains our own destiny. Agreeing with Pablo Picasso who said, "I don't develop; I am.," Hillman believes the "soul's code" is written on our hearts from the beginning and that life is an opportunity to express, with increasing authenticity, that which we essentially are. Hillman encourages us to give ourselves to our destiny, to "recognize the call as a prime fact of human existence" and to "align life with it." He reminds us, "A calling may be postponed, avoided, intermittently missed. It may possess you completely. Whatever; eventually it will out. It makes its claim. The daimon does not go away" (p. 6).

I would like to add my own testimony to these voices. My daimon was to be an artist--a writer and poet. But all my life I fought this artistic calling. Raised in a rural, isolated area, I had no one to tell me about art, creativity, and the world of imagination. Yet I was always drawn to this world, always knew at some level that it was my destiny. When I decided to become a minister, my daimon was at work, drawing me to a profession where I could feel, at times, the numinous. Later, when I became a psychologist, I was responding to this same pull of destiny. For me, psychology was a way to explore the deep poetic soul. From the start I was drawn to the humanistic and existential perspectives, never to the medical and mechanistic, because I saw in the former the imaginative depth and creative possibilities I craved. But both the ministry and psychology were only approximations, stations on the way. They were substitutes for a whole-hearted response to the call of destiny.

Then, at midlife, the call became more insistent. My defenses began breaking down. I cried the first time I read Rumi's (1984) poem that says:

> Inside you there's an artist
> you don't know about...
> Is what I say true? Say yes quickly,
> if you know, if you've known it
> from the beginning of the universe. (p. 69)

I was 49 when I finally saw with clarity the destiny I had avoided. I shrank back, afraid. I wrote in my journal, "It's taken me 49 years to know who I am, and now I fear I'm too old to be it. What do I do with the accumulations of what I'm not? Can an older body contain the passions of new dreams? Can I start at the beginning again and honor that young boy who, with the best of intentions, went down so many wrong roads?"

I have now learned the answers to those questions: It is never too late to go to Nineveh, never too late to be coughed up onto the shores of one's destiny. Older bodies *can* contain the passion of new dreams. New wine does not burst old wineskins; it makes them moist, supple, and strong. One can always start again, must always start again.

So, after many years of resisting, I finally listened to my daimon and took the plunge. I began to write and even, in time, to think of myself as a writer, poet, and artist. When asked my profession, instead of saying "psychologist" or "professor," I sometimes found the courage to say "writer" or even "poet." I still feel embarrassed by those designations, afraid that I am not worthy to be called by those titles. Perhaps this is how it is with destiny. We know that this is serious business, the stuff of "ultimate concerns."

When we give ourselves to destiny, we feel tremendous awe and great humility. This is not ego, not some grandiose delusion about "our gift" or "saving the world." Rather this is the quiet celebration of a heart that has finally found itself; it is the tearful humility of a prodigal soul that has finally come home.

The daimon is always playing its flute out there on the mountain. The soul is always calling, singing her gentle song of homecoming. But we continue going "up and down the earth" doing what we feel we must, hanging back, buying time. But destiny waits, unbearably patient, increasingly insistent, until one day we finally give up, give in, and go home to the only place we were ever meant to be--the place of personal destiny which James Joyce (1964) called "near to the wild heart of life." (p. 171)

Nothing is more important than being true to ourselves, to the daimon that lives at the core of our soul. And what if this means that we walk alone, that no one understands, that no one knows our name? Rilke (1989) gives us the answer:

> And if the earthly no longer knows your name,
> whisper to the silent earth: I'm flowing.
> To the flashing water say: I am. (p. 255)

Conclusion

I would like to end with two poems that express my alternative vision. The first is by D. H. Lawrence (1977) and is called *Healing*.

> I am not a mechanism, an
>   assembly of various sections
> And it is not because the mechanism
>   is working wrongly that I am ill
> I am ill because of wounds to the soul
>   to the deep emotional self
> And the wounds to the soul
>   take a long, long time
> Only time can help
>   and patience
> And a certain difficult repentance,

Long, difficult repentance,
Realization of life's mistake,
And the freeing oneself from the
      endless repetition of the mistake
Which mankind at large has
      chosen to sanctify. (p. 620)

The second poem is called *Leonard.* I wrote this poem a few years ago. It points to an alternative and more compassionate way of viewing the suffering client.

They shot Leonard full of thorazene
But still he banged his bleeding head
Against the wailing wall
Of the lock-up room
His cries of "God have mercy!"
Filling the halls
And keeping everyone awake.
Then they tried behavior mod:
Ten minutes of walking the grounds
For every hour Leonard was banging free
It worked for awhile
Leonard spent some nice summer days
Counting the bricks on the west wall (96,463)
And giving the attendant a high five
Every time the resident peacock spread its tail.
But by summer's end, Leonard was banging again
Skinner, it seemed, had hit a wall

In October they gave him electroshock
"Last resort," the psychiatrist said.
"That banging could damage his brain"
(Irony was not a word he learned in medical school)
After three treatments the banging stopped.
Even Leonard himself was so shocked by the results
That he lay in bed for two weeks in a catatonic stupor
Apparently contemplating the miracles of modern medicine
But by November 10 he was banging again
Faster and harder now, making up for lost time

When Myra, the intern, came
They gave her an orientation to the ward
Which included watching Leonard bang his head
Not yet skilled in medical ways
Myra touched Leonard's shoulder.
"I wish you wouldn't bang your head like that," she said.
"It hurts my heart to watch"
Leonard kept on banging but when she left the room
He stopped long enough to gaze after her
A look of amazement on his face…

When I was a graduate student, the professors who damaged me most were those who had such "good boundaries," as we say, that I always felt like an object on the other side of their walls. I find it puzzling that in other areas of society we condemn those who treat others as objects, but in psychology we not only continue to treat others as objects but we invent jargon such as "good boundaries" and "blank screens" to justify our aloofness and unavailability. Here's what I believe: anything we do that diminishes our clients' or our students' humanity is unethical.

When the spirit of compassion dies, its remains are embalmed in the form of an ethical code.

Appendix

Why I Left Psychology (Almost): A Fictional Story That Might Be True

Overview: This fictional, humorous story pokes fun at one of our profession's sacred cows and raises fundamental questions about our increasingly legalistic approach to ethics. The intent is not to make fun of genuine professional ethics but to point to a deeper, more sophisticated understanding of this important topic. The story is entirely fictional and the characters and settings are not real. However, if you think you recognize some of the characters in the story, perhaps even yourself, you could be right because the chapter is indeed "a fictional story that might be true."

Introduction

This introduction provides a scholarly frame for the fictional story that follows. The English word "ethics" comes from roots that have to do with one's character, yet in psychology we increasingly use the term as a synonym for "rules of conduct" in the profession.

Far too often those who teach "law and ethics" courses in graduate psychology programs and in continuing education classes focus on the many rules of the ethics code and spend little time discussing ethics per se. I fear we are training psychologists to be legalists instead of ethical professionals who know how to apply wisdom, compassion, and justice to the complex situations they confront as psychologists.

Years ago Kohlberg (1976) and Gilligan (1982) made us aware that there are different levels of moral development and functioning. Kohlberg (1976) posited a hierarchy of moral development that viewed legalistic rule-keeping as a sign of lower-level moral functioning and following high-level moral principles as the ideal. Gilligan (1982) pointed out limitations of Kohlberg's research and model and emphasized that a true "ethic of care" is not simply about following an abstract moral principle--even a worthy one--but more about compassionately considering all those who will be affected by a particular action or decision. Kohlberg and Gilligan did agree, however, that there are degrees or levels of moral functioning and that legalistic adherence to rules represents a lower level of such functioning. In my fictional story readers will hear the echoes of Kohlberg and Gilligan.

In regard to the ethics of dual relationships, an issue addressed in my fictional story, Lazarus and Zur (2002) raised concerns about our profession's negative attitude toward all dual relationships and argued that *certain* carefully considered multiple relationships with clients can be not only ethical but highly beneficial. Their thoughtful, scholarly approach to this complex issue is a breath of fresh air in a profession where legalistic attitudes seem to be gaining ground and where it is sometimes difficult to determine how much of our ethical thinking is driven by genuine concern for clients and how much is driven simply by fear of lawsuits. To avoid giving the wrong message, however, I would like to make it clear that I am not advocating that psychologists and clients (or professors and students) should be free to engage in any kind of dual relationship they wish. Indeed, certain dual relationships can be problematic, damaging, even disastrous. For example, I believe that sexual involvements with current clients or students should always be avoided. Having made that clear, however, I do agree with Lazarus and Zur that our profession has swung too far in the other direction, having become paranoid about all dual relationships and having failed to see the benefits of carefully considered multiple involvements, along with the very real damage that too much "professional distance" can do. I hope my fictional story will shed light on these issues.

Although I said my story is "entirely fictional," one small part is true. I actually was a conservative minister and left the church more than 30 years ago. My theological training involved a strong dose of ethics and one of the first lessons I learned as a young ministerial student was that ethics and rules are not the same. Genuine ethics has to do with the development of a just and compassionate human being. Rules, on the other hand, are the province of legalists who tend to become more concerned about rule-keeping than about what it means to be a truly good human being.

Regarding my personal views on the opinions expressed in the fictional story, I agree with all those who challenged the young professor in this sense: They were all at least intuitively aware that genuine ethics involves more than simply applying a black and white rule from an ethics code. I especially identify with the grandmotherly woman crocheting the afghan who took it upon herself to point out the difference between legalism and genuine ethics. She expressed my point of view beautifully--far better than I could have done myself.

Finally, just for the record: In my long career as a clinical psychologist and professor, I have never been accused of an ethical violation nor was I ever the object of a lawsuit. The only way I can account for this is that I had very forgiving clients and students.

I hope you enjoy the following story and find that its humorous, fictional nature does not dim its illumination of a very serious topic.

The Story

Awhile back I had reached the end of my rope with psychology. I was angry as hell and I wasn't going to take it anymore. I hated HMOs, clerks with B.S. degrees telling me how and when I could treat my clients, APA formulating treatment guidelines to tell me how to practice, short-term therapies being taught to our graduate students so they can get jobs in the insane marketplace, psychologists seeking prescription privileges as though we don't have enough pill-pushers in this country as it is, and colleagues all around me using models of therapy that would work better with rats and pigeons than with human beings. I'll admit it: I was one cynical S.O.B. I had talked it over with my wife and was making plans to refer my clients. As soon as the task was accomplished properly, I planned to turn in my license and do something more honorable such as selling used cars or working as a telemarketer.

But you don't know me from Adam, so let me back up and tell you a little about myself. I became a psychologist in 1973. For thirty years I've listened to clients' hopes and dreams. I've witnessed their courage in the face of tragedy and loss. I've watched middle-aged men who had lost their way find their souls again. I've seen abused women rise up and become strong. I've seen little boys and girls, depressed by burdens no child should have to bear, find joy again. I've seen marginalized people find their voice and become forces for change. I wouldn't trade these experiences for anything in the world. Nevertheless, I was going to turn in my license and leave the profession.

It wouldn't have been the first time I had bailed out of a profession. I grew up in the Bible belt and was originally trained as a fundamentalist minister back in the 1960s. After five years of giving it my best, I knew I wasn't cut out for the job. No matter how hard I tried, I couldn't follow all the rules and I felt like a hypocrite. I'd preach against lust but find myself staring at the shapely bodies of female parishioners in the church parking lot as soon as church was over. I'd tell my parishioners to read the Bible every day, but I didn't do it myself. The truth is, I found the Bible pretty dull, especially those Old Testament passages about who begat whom and those stories about how God commanded his people to wipe out whole towns including the women and children. I found that hard to swallow. Also, I sometimes found it hard to pray for the sick, especially those who were obviously dying. I remember going to the hospital to visit a man in his thirties who was eaten up with cancer. In six months, he had gone from 175 pounds to 85. He had a wife and two young kids who loved him more than anything else in the world. When I arrived, his wife took me aside and asked if I would beseech God for her husband's life. She used the word *beseech* because she thought it meant to beg God with everything in you. I knew her husband was going to die and there wasn't anything I could do about it, but when I saw the desperation in her eyes, I walked over to the bed, took the man's bony hand, and I beseeched God--as best I could --to let this young husband and father live. He died two days later.

I think that's when I decided to leave the ministry. I wasn't good enough and didn't believe enough to be a man of God. I couldn't follow all the rules, and I didn't have enough faith to save anyone. My family and I lived in Michigan at the time so I resigned from the ministry and took a job on the Fisher Body assembly line. My wife was with me all the way, but when my parents and the rest of my clan heard that I had left the ministry, they thought I was going crazy. I thought I was becoming sane.

It took me about a week to know I didn't want to build cars the rest of my life. I still wanted to help people. A friend asked me if I had ever considered becoming a psychologist. "Not really," I said. But after thinking about it for a couple of days, I thought it might work. Psychology was a secular profession and maybe it didn't have a bunch of rules and maybe you could serve others even if you weren't perfect. With a renewed sense of hope, I applied to a doctoral psychology program on the East Coast. To my surprise, they accepted me and I began classes in the fall of 1969. Almost immediately, I felt at home. I knew I had found my place in the world. Humanistic psychology was at its peak and almost every class I took, regardless of its title, turned into an encounter group where students and professors talked heart-to-heart. We didn't know about the horrible dangers of dual relationships in those days. We went to our professors' homes, drank beer with them at the local pizza place, and discussed everything from the sexual revolution to the heavy social issues of that time. My doctoral class of fifteen students was made up of whites, blacks, Jews, Latinos, Asians, and, of course, one former fundamentalist minister. We argued, got angry, cried, supported each other, and somehow found a way to stick together. One of our professors owned a cabin in upstate New York and once during spring break we all piled into cars and spent the week with him and his wife at their place in the mountains. I could not have received a better education.

One of my classmates, a bright Latino woman whom we all adored, was working at the university clinic. She fell in love with one of her male clients and he fell in love right back at her. She discussed this openly in our practicum class and tried, unsuccessfully, to work through her feelings. Ultimately, she decided her feelings were real and not simply countertransference. Our practicum professor, an elderly man who was both wise and kind, told her she must bring the therapy to an end, make sure the young man was properly referred to another therapist, and then he saw no reason they couldn't date. The young woman handled the situation beautifully. A year later she and her former client were married. Today, they have three grown children and four grandchildren. I attended their thirtieth wedding anniversary last August and they're still madly in love with each other.

During the second year of my doctoral program, I had a group therapy class with a wonderful professor. When the course came to an end, I asked her if she would take me as a client. She said that if I didn't plan to take any more classes with her, she would be glad to see me in therapy. Since I was a graduate psychology student, she asked if I would like to serve as a co-therapist in one of the therapy groups she ran at her clinic. I jumped at the chance. I had my personal therapy with her on Tuesday mornings and then I'd help her run the therapy group on Tuesday nights. My group work often brought up issues for me that I would discuss in my personal therapy. She was my support system through the rest of my doctoral program and wrote me a glowing letter of recommendation that helped me land a top-notch internship. Through my multiple relationships with this brilliant and caring woman, I gained confidence and maturity as both a person and a professional. I completed my internship after a year and graduated in 1972 with my PhD in clinical psychology. A year later I passed the state licensing exam and in 1973 five of my classmates and I, along with one of our favorite professors who was retiring from the university, started a clinic. Our beloved professor died in 1994, but the rest of us still work together at the same clinic. We estimate that we have served more than 20,000 clients over the past thirty years.

Fortunately, none of us has ever been sued and only one of us--a man whom I'll call John--has ever been accused of an ethical violation. A little over a year ago, John was working with a female client who began showing up at our clinic at odd times and demanding to be seen. After rearranging his schedule a couple of times to accommodate her, he finally told her that, unless it was a true emergency, she would have to stick with her regular appointments and that he would not see her any more on a "walk-in" basis. A few days later the client sent a letter to the state psychology board saying that John had "abandoned" her and that if they didn't revoke his license, she would sue both John and the board. The board took nearly a year to investigate the matter. The five-member committee interrogated John on two different occasions for more than two hours each time. John had to get colleagues to write letters on his behalf and he consulted his attorney numerous times while the investigation was going on. Finally, after a year the psychology board decided the allegation was groundless and dismissed the charge. Of course, John's life had been disrupted and he had been pushed to the brink of depression, worrying and trying to defend himself against a ridiculous charge. John is one of the kindest, most ethical people I know. It was hard to see him go through that.

For me, John's ordeal was the last straw. As I said earlier, I was already disillusioned with my profession so it was easy to decide to quit. However, because the expiration date of my psychology license was coming up soon, I knew I'd have to renew it in order to have time to end with my clients. That meant I'd have to finish my continuing education units required to renew my license. Ironically, the one CE class I still needed was "Law and Ethics."

The "Law and Ethics" class, which was offered as a one-day workshop in a nearby city, was taught by a young professor who had gotten his doctorate a couple of years before at a well-known school on the West Coast. As he began the class, he told us quite proudly that he had always wanted to be a lawyer but had decided at the last minute to become a psychologist instead. With that introduction, he launched into what would turn out to be a seven-hour lecture, with a lunch break in the middle, focused mainly on the ethics code of the American Psychological Association.

The young professor had a way with words and with his lawyer-like mind he managed to ferret out nuances from the ethics code that I had never even considered. He peppered his lecture with case illustrations to show how easily--and sometimes without even knowing it--one could become an unethical psychologist. He handled questions from the audience with ease, giving thorough and crystal-clear answers. At one point he was talking about the requirement in the ethics code that psychology training programs must tell students before entering the program if they will be expected to discuss personal information as part of their training. An old professor sitting next to me raised his hand. "Are you telling me," he asked, "that I could be brought up on ethical charges if I ask students in my group psychotherapy class to share something personal about themselves-- even if I make it clear that they can share at whatever level they wish?" The young professor smiled benevolently across the forty years that separated him from the old gentleman. "Let's put it this way," he said, with just a touch of condescension, "If your university has not officially informed students when they applied to the program that they could be asked to share personal information in some classes, then you would be ethically at risk if you were to ask your students to reveal anything of a personal nature." The old gentleman shook his head in disbelief and went back to doodling on his notepad, but I heard him say under his breath, "What the hell do they think psychology is about anyway?"

The professor continued his exegesis of the ethics code. By the time we broke for lunch, I had counted thirteen violations I was quite sure I had committed and thirty-three others that were real possibilities. I was scared and having fundamentalist flashbacks. The professor reminded me of ministers I knew as a boy who seemed to enjoy naming all the sins one could commit that would send you to hell. I flashed back to my ministerial training and to the famous sermon by Jonathan Edwards titled "Sinners in the Hands of an Angry God." Members of his congregation had actually fainted when Edwards described in graphic language how sinners dangle by nothing but a thread over the fires of hell. After listening to the young professor, I knew that I was dangling by a thread over the fires of psychology hell and my only hope was that my clients would be nice enough not to turn me in. What scared me most--which also reminded me of my fundamentalist upbringing--was that ignorance and good intentions made no difference. The young professor had made it clear: if we violated the ethics code, we would be cast into hell and nobody --certainly not the American Psychological Association--would come to our rescue.

I went to a fast food restaurant for lunch and had a sourdough burger and a large diet coke. Fast food always calms my nerves so by the time I returned for the afternoon session, I was feeling better and thought maybe I had simply overreacted. Little did I know that the worst was yet to come. The afternoon session focused on multiple relationships and the young professor described in great detail all the sins one could commit related to such relationships. For example, he told us in no uncertain terms that we were putting ourselves at grievous ethical risk if we became friends with a client when therapy ended. He said that while the ethics code did not explicitly address this issue, almost all problems between therapists and former clients had begun with such "boundary violations." A woman at the back of the audience who was crocheting a purple afghan and wearing beads she had apparently salvaged from the 1960s pointed out that this was strange since the ethics code allowed therapists, if certain stringent criteria were met, to date a former client two years after therapy ended. Holding the afghan up to inspect her work, she asked the young professor nonchalantly, "Does that mean I can have sex with a client after two years so long as we don't become friends?" The audience cracked up. We thought she was pretty funny. The young professor didn't. "Are you making fun of the ethics code?" he asked, with a sternness that reminded me of Jerry Falwell. "Of course not," said the woman as she began crocheting again. "I would never poke fun at a sacred cow."

The young professor didn't quite know what to say. After all, the woman was old enough to be his grandmother and judging by the laughter, the class seemed to be on her side. So he cleared his throat and took up where he had left off, forging ahead to describe more perils of multiple relationships.

"Suppose your client owns a car dealership in town," he said, "and you are in the market for a new car. Should you buy your car from your client or should you go somewhere else?"

An attractive young woman sitting on the front row asked quickly, "Current client or past client?"

The professor smiled. I got the feeling he liked the young woman. She had wild blonde hair, wore tight blue jeans, and had a body that would stop a train–not that I had noticed, of course.

"Let's say for sake of argument that he's a current client," replied the professor.

"Then no way," said the young woman. "If you bought a car from him, it could mess up the transference big time."

"Ding!" said the professor. "You get an 'A' in my class."

The young woman smiled. She had nice lips and perfect white teeth. "Why thank you, Professor," she said in a coy voice that somehow reminded me of Britney Spears. I couldn't help but wonder if we were witnessing a dual relationship in-the-making. To be honest, I was feeling a little old and jealous. At that moment I would have been glad to see the handsome young professor dangle over hell and even drop--as long as he left Britney behind.

"Now, let's make it more difficult," said the professor. For a moment, I thought we were about to go deep. I was wrong. "Suppose the car dealer's therapy had ended a year ago. Would it be okay for you to buy a car from him?"

This was obviously too complex a question for Britney. Besides her score was perfect so far, and I had the feeling she didn't want to mess it up by saying something stupid.

A man sitting across the aisle from me--I'd say he was in his early forties--raised his hand. "Generally speaking, I think it would be okay," he said. "I worked in a small town in South Carolina for ten years and actually faced this problem. One of my clients was the local car dealer--the only dealer for miles around. He came to see me for about a year. I bought one car from him when he was my client and a couple of others through the years after he ended therapy. I can't see that it hurt anything. In fact, I think he would have been upset with me if I hadn't bought from him."

The young professor nodded. He had decided to try a more understanding approach. "Well, in the old days," he said, "such loose ethics were quite common, especially in small towns. But if you lived there today, what would be the ethical thing to do?"

The man looked a little put-out with the professor. I figured the term "old days" or maybe "loose ethics" is what had riled him. "Well, I guess I'd just have to forget ethics and do the right thing," he said with a rising voice and a heavy Southern accent I hadn't noticed before. "I'd buy my cars from him just like I always did and I'd also have him over for supper if I wanted to!"

This was a pretty direct challenge to the professor's authority and several of us sat up in our seats to see what would happen. The professor was red-faced and the veins on his perfectly tanned neck were standing out. For a minute I thought he was going to jump over desks and tear the man's heart out. Instead, he pointed his well-manicured finger at the man--and at all of us dangling sinners, I thought. "Listen to me," he said. "Some of the best minds in our profession wrote these ethical standards. They are designed to guide us, protect us, and keep us from being sued. If you want to ignore them or make fun of them, then go ahead, but remember this: You will end up before an ethics committee, very possibly lose your license, and be personally and professionally humiliated and disgraced." By the time he finished, the young professor was almost shouting. I was having a panic attack and had slouched down in my seat waiting for an angel of God to swoop down and cut the threads of those of us who were dangling over hell because of multiple relationships with car dealers.

The woman with the afghan didn't seem particularly perturbed. "I always thought ethics was about love, compassion, and making sure we treated our clients with dignity and respect," she said, her quiet voice in stark contrast to the professor's loud ranting that still hung in the room. "Unfortunately, classes like this, along with those we get in graduate school, always seem to focus on rules--and rules don't have much to do with ethics, really."

Everybody became quiet. The woman continued. "I wonder how many of those who wrote the ethics code have formal training in ethics. And what about those who teach ethics in our graduate programs and in continuing education classes like this one? If I were to guess, I'd say very few have formal training in ethical thought. Ethics is a huge and complex field. I have two doctorates, one in philosophy with a specialization in ethics and one in clinical psychology. The program in ethics was much more difficult than the psychology program."

She looked at the professor and gave him a grandmotherly smile. "You seem like a nice young man," she said, not a trace of condescension in her voice. "But let me ask you: do you have any formal training in ethics?"

The professor stammered. "Well, I... I ... I have spent my entire professional life studying law and ethics in psychology," he said.

"I'm sure you have," said the woman, "and you are very bright and articulate. But based on what I've heard here today, I'd say you're a legalist--one who knows all the rules but little about ethics."

At this point I was getting intrigued and had even stopped watching for swooping angels.

The woman continued, "Legalism is an old problem when it comes to ethics. People start out with good intentions. They know that compassion and justice are important, so they attempt to capture these qualities in a written code. It never works because people begin to focus on the rules and forget about the values that gave rise to the rules in the first place. Genuine ethics can never be captured in a list of rules, no matter how detailed. In fact, rules tend to kill compassion and justice. As one of my philosophy professors used to say, 'When the spirit of compassion dies, its remains are embalmed in the form of an ethical code.'"

She paused for a moment to let that sink in, and then continued, "And why do we have all these detailed rules about multiple relationships? That kind of tediousness is rather new in psychology and I suspect it came about primarily due to lawsuits, not good ethical thinking. Certainly, we must never exploit or damage our clients through multiple relationships, or in any other way. The same is true of professor-student relationships. I'm a professor, so let me speak to that. The legalists in our profession seem so concerned about personal sharing and multiple levels of connection between professors and students. Of course, we all know professors who have exploited students, just as we know unscrupulous therapists who have taken advantage of clients. But just because we have unethical professionals among us who use personal connections and open sharing to exploit students and clients, does this mean that personal connections and open sharing are therefore inherently suspect? What kind of twisted thinking leads us to such ridiculous conclusions?"

She looked up from her crocheting to see if anyone cared to answer her rhetorical question. When no one said anything, she continued. "And then there's the ethical issue that no one ever seems to address: What damage is done when we are so concerned about multiple relationships that we never go to lunch with our students, never invite them to our homes, never interact with them anywhere except in the cold environs of classrooms and faculty offices? Or what does it do to the soul of a student who speaks of something personal in class and is then told by the professor, explicitly or implicitly, that such topics are not appropriate in the classroom. What message does this send to students about opening up their hearts, about becoming warmer and more compassionate human beings? What message does it give our students about how to treat their own students when they become professors? As an ethicist, I find it strange that no one in psychology seems to be asking about the damage that emotionally unavailable professors do, not to mention emotionally unavailable therapists whose name is legion. When I was a graduate student, the professors who damaged me most were those who had such "good boundaries," as we say, that I always felt like an object on the other side of their walls. I find it puzzling that in other areas of society we condemn those who treat others as objects but in psychology we not only continue to treat others as objects but we invent jargon such as "good boundaries" and "blank screens" to justify our aloofness and unavailability. Here's what I believe: Anything we do that diminishes our clients' or our students' humanity is unethical."

The woman stopped and the room was silent. Her last sentence seemed to hang in the air. *Anything we do that diminishes our clients' or our students' humanity is unethical.* We were in the presence of wisdom and we knew it. Some of us, reminded of more humane times in our profession, had tears in our eyes. Even Britney and the young professor were quiet. I wasn't sure either of them had actually gotten the point, but at least they knew when to be silent. Finally, someone noticed the time and said, "It's 5 o'clock. Time to go." We all got up and filed silently out of the room, picking up our CE certificates on our way out the door.

When I got home, my wife was in the yard tending the roses.

"How'd your class go?" she asked. "Was it as boring as you predicted?"

"No, it actually turned out to be pretty good," I said.

For some reason, I wanted to break through boundaries, so I walked over and gave her a hug. "Honey, I think I'll stay at the clinic after all," I said. "Would that be okay with you?"

"Of course," she said. "I was hoping you wouldn't quit. I know how much you love what you do."

I smiled but didn't say anything. I went in the house and began making phone calls to some old colleagues and clients--just to tell them how much they meant to me.

About the Author

David N. Elkins, PhD, is a licensed clinical psychologist, a Professor Emeritus of psychology in the Graduate School of Education and Psychology, Pepperdine University, and a member of the Core Faculty at the School of Professional Psychology, University of the Rockies. Dr. Elkins is on the editorial boards of three professional journals and has served as president of Division 32, Society for Humanistic Psychology, of the American Psychological Association. He has helped train clinical psychologists for 25 years. He lives in Colorado with his wife, Sara, and a Yorkie named "Peanuts."

References

Aanstoos, C. Serlin, I., & Greening, T. (2000). History of Division 32 (Humanistic Psychology) of the American Psychology Association. In D. Dewsbuty (Ed.), *Unification through division: Histories of the Divisions of the American Psychological Association*, (Vol. V; pp. 85-112). Washington, DC: American Psychological Association.

Adler, A. (1929). *The science of living*. New York: Doubleday.

Adler, A. (1930). *The education of children*. Chicago: Henry Regnery.

Adler, A. (1931). *What life should mean to you*. New York: Putnam.

Ahn, H. & Wampold, B.E. (2001). Where oh where are the specific ingredients? A meta-analysis of component studies in counseling and psychotherapy. *Journal of Counseling Psychology, 48*, 251-257.

American Psychiatric Association. (2000). *Diagnostic and statistical manual of mental disorders* (4th ed., text rev.). Washington, DC: Author.

Anderson, W. T. (Ed.). (1990). *Reality isn't what it used to be*. San Francisco, CA: Harper Collins.

Anderson, W. T. (1998). *The future of self: Inventing the postmodern person*. Los Angeles, CA: Tarcher.

APA Presidential Task Force on Evidence-Based Practice (2006). Evidence-based practice in psychology. *American Psychologist, 61*(4), 271-285.

Apfelbaum, B. & Apfelbaum, C. (1973). Encountering encounter groups: A reply to Koch and Haigh. *Journal of Humanistic Psychology, 13*, 53-67.

Arbuckle, D. S. (1973). Koch's distortion of encounter group theory. *Journal of Humanistic Psychology, 13*, 47-51.

Arons, M. (1994). Creativity, humanistic psychology, and the American zeitgeist. In F. Wertz (Ed.), *The humanistic movement* (pp. 45-61). Lake Worth, FL: Gardner.

Arons, M. & Richards, R. (2001). Two noble insurgencies: Creativity and humanistic psychology. In K. J. Schneider, J. F. T. Bugental, & J. Frasier (Eds.), *The handbook of humanistic psychology* (pp. 127-142). Thousand Oaks, CA: Sage.

Asay, T. P. & Lambert, M. J. (1999). The empirical case for the common factors in psychotherapy. In M.A. Hubble, B. L. Duncan, & S. D. Miller (Eds.), *The heart and soul of change* (pp. 23-55). Washington, DC: American Psychological Association.

Barrett-Lennard, G. T. (1998). *Carl Rogers' helping system: Journey and substance.* Thousand Oaks: Sage.

Bellah, R. N., Madsen, R., Sullivan, W. M., Swidler, A., & Tipton, S. M. (1985*). Habits of the heart: Individualism and commitment in American life.* Berkeley, CA: University of California Press.

Benish, S. G., Imel, Z. E., & Wampold, B. E. (2008). The relative efficacy of bona fide psychotherapies for treating post-traumatic stress disorder: A meta-analysis of direct comparisons. *Clinical Psychology Review, 28*(5), 746-758.

Bennett, F. D. (1976). Encounter groups: Growth or addiction? *Journal of Humanistic Psychology, 16*(4) 59-70.

Bergin, A. E. (1971). The evaluation of therapeutic outcomes. In A. E. Bergin & S.L. Garfield (Eds.), *Handbook of psychotherapy and behavior change* (pp. 217-270). New York: Wiley.

Bergin, A. E. (1997). Neglect of the therapist and the human dimensions of change: A commentary. *Clinical Psychology: Science and Practice, 4*, 83-89.

Bergin, A. E., & Lambert, M. J. (1978). The evaluation of outcomes in psychotherapy. In A. E. Bergin & S. L. Garfield (Eds.) *Handbook of psychotherapy and behavior change* (pp. 217-270). New York: Wiley.

Bloom, B. L. (1992). *Planned short-term psychotherapy: A clinical handbook.* Boston: Allyn and Bacon

Bobgan, M. & Bobgan, D. (1989). *Prophets of psychoheresy II.* Santa Barbara, CA: Eastgate Publishers.

Bohart, A. & Tallman, K. (1996). The active client: Therapy as self-help. *Journal of Humanistic Psychology, 36*, 7-30.

Bohart, A. & Tallman, K. (1999) *How clients make therapy work: The process of active self-healing.* Washington, DC: American Psychological Association.

Bozarth, J. D., Zimring, F. M., & Tausch, R. (2001). Client-centered therapy: The evolution of a revolution. In D. J. Cain and J. Seeman (Eds.), *Humanistic psychotherapies:*

Handbook of research and practice (pp. 147-188). Washington, DC: American Psychological Association.

Breggin, P. (1991). *Toxic psychiatry: Why empathy, therapy and love must replace the drugs, electroshock and biochemical theories of the "new psychiatry."* New York: St. Martin's Press.

Breuer, J. & Freud, S. (1893-1895). *Studies on hysteria, Vol. II of The Standard Edition of the Complete Psychological Works of Sigmund Freud.* London: Hogarth Press, 1955.

Brome, V. (1981). *Jung: Man and myth.* New York: Atheneum Books.

Brownback, P. (1982). *The danger of self-love.* Chicago, IL: Moody Press.

Budman, S. H. & Gurman, A. S. (1983). The practice of brief therapy. *Professional Psychology: Research and Practice, 14,* 277-292.

Budman, S. H. & Gurman, A. S. (1988). *The theory and practice of brief therapy.* New York: Guilford Press.

Bugental, J. F. T. (1976). *The search for existential identity.* San Francisco: Jossey-Bass.

Bugental, J. F. T. (1981). *The search for authenticity.* New York: Irvington.

Bugental, J. F. T. & Bracke, P. E. (1992). The future of humanistic-existential psychotherapy. *Psychotherapy, 29*(1), 28-33.

Burns, D. (1999). *Feeling good: The new mood therapy.* New York: Harper Collins.

Burns, D. & Nolen-Hoeksema, S. (1992). Therapeutic empathy and recovery from depression in cognitive-behavioral therapy: A structural equation model. *Journal of Consulting and Clinical Psychology, 60,* 441-449.

Buss, A. R. (1979). Humanistic psychology as liberal ideology: The socio-historical roots of Maslow's theory of self-actualization. *Journal of Humanistic Psychology, 19*(3), 43-55.

Cain, D. J. (2003). Advancing humanistic psychology and psychotherapy: Some challenges and proposed solutions. *Journal of Humanistic Psychology, 43*(3), 10-41.

Cain, D. J. (2001a). Defining characteristics, history, and evolution of humanistic psychotherapies. In D. J. Cain & J. Seeman (Eds.), *Humanistic psychotherapies: Handbook of research and practice* (pp. 3-54). Washington, DC: American Psychological Association.

Cain, D. J. (2001b). Preface. In D. J. Cain & J. Seeman (Eds.), *Humanisti psychotherapies: Handbook of research and practice* (pp. 147-188). Washington, DC: American Psychological Association.

Cain, D. J. & Seeman, J. (Eds.). (2002). *Humanistic psychotherapies: Handbook of research and practice.* Washington, DC: APA Books.

Castonguay, L. G. (1993). "Common factors" and "nonspecific variables": Clarification of the two concepts and recommendations for research. *Journal of Psychotherapy Integration, 3,* 267-286.

Consumer Reports. (1995, November). Mental health: Does therapy help? pp. 734-739.

DeCarvalho, R. J. (1991*). The founders of humanistic psychology.* New York: Praeger.

Dublin, J. E. (1972). Whose image of what? Open letter to Sigmund Koch. *Journal of Humanistic Psychology, 12,* 79-85.

Durkheim, E. (1915). *The elementary forms of religious life.* London: George, Allen and Unwin.

Dush, D. M., Hirt, M. L., & Schroeder, H. (1983). Self-statement modification with adults: A meta-analysis. *Journal of Consulting and Clinical Psychology, 94,* 408-422.

Eisenberg, D. M., Davis, R. B., Ettner, S. L., Appel, S., Wilkey, S., Van Rompay, M., & Kessler, R. C. (1998). Trends in alternative medicine use in the United States, 1990-1997. *Journal of the American Medical Association, 280,* 1569-1575.

Eliade, M. (1961). *The sacred and the profane.* New York: Harper & Row.

Elkins, D. (1997). My old Jungian analyst. *Journal of Humanistic Psychology, 38* (1), 41.

Elkins, D. N. (1998). *Beyond religion: A personal program for building a spiritual life outside the walls of traditional religion.* Wheaton, IL: Quest Books.

Elkins, D. N. (2000). Old Saybrook I and II: The visioning and revisioning of humanistic psychology. *Journal of Humanistic Psychology, 40*(2), 119-127.

Elkins, D. N. (2001). Beyond religion: Toward a humanistic spirituality. In K. J. Schneider, J. F. T. Bugental, & J. Frasier (Eds.), *The handbook of humanistic psychology* (pp. 201-212), Thousand Oaks, CA: Sage.

Elkins, D. N. (2004). The deep poetic soul: An alternative vision of psychotherapy. *The Humanistic Psychologist 32*(4), 76-102.

Elkins, D. N. (2006). Why I left psychology (almost): A fictional story that might be true. *The Humanistic Psychologist 34*(2), 99-109.

Elkins, D. N. (2007). Empirically supported treatments: The deconstruction of a myth. *Journal of Humanistic Psychology, 47*(4), 474-500.

Elkins, D. N. (2008). Short-term, linear approaches to psychotherapy: What we now know. *Journal of Humanistic Psychology, 48*(3) 413-431.

Elkins, D. N. (2009a). The medical model in psychotherapy: Its limitations and failures. *Journal of Humanistic Psychology, 49*(1), 66-84.

Elkins, D. N. (2009b). Why humanistic psychology lost its power and influence in American psychology: Implications for advancing humanistic psychology. *Journal of Humanistic Psychology, 49*(3), 267-291.

Elliott, R. (2002). Research on the effectiveness of humanistic therapies: A meta-analysis. In D. Cain & J. Seeman (Eds.), *Humanistic psychotherapies: Handbook of research and practice* (pp. 57-82). Washington, DC: American Psychological Association.

Elliott, R., Greenberg, L.S., & Litaer, G. (2003). In A. E. Bergin & S. L. Garfield (Eds.), *Handbook of psychotherapy and behavior change* (pp. 493-540), New York: Wiley.

Epel, N. (1993). *Writers dreaming.* New York: Vintage Books.

Fox, D. & Prilleltensky, I. (1997). *Critical Psychology: An Introduction.* London: Sage.

Frank, J. D. & Frank, J. B. (1991). *Persuasion and healing: A comparative study of psychotherapy* (3rd ed.) Baltimore, MD: Johns Hopkins University Press.

Frankl, V. (1963). *Man's search for meaning.* New York: Simon & Schuster.

Frankl. V. (1978). *The unheard cry for meaning: Psychotherapy and humanism.* New York: Simon & Schuster.

Frankl, V. (1986). *The doctor and the soul.* New York: Random.

Friedman, M. (1976). Aiming at the self: The paradox of encounter and the human potential movement. *Journal of Humanistic Psychology, 16,* 5-34.

Gendlin, E. T. (1992). Celebrations and problems of humanistic psychology. *The Humanistic Psychologist, 20*(2-3), 447-460.

Gilligan, C. (1982). *In a different voice.* Cambridge, MA: Harvard University Press.

Giorgi, A. (1968). Existential phenomenology and the psychology of the human person. *Review of Existential Psychology and Psychiatry, 8,* 102-116.

Giorgi, A. (1970). *Psychology as a human science.* New York: Harper & Row.

Giorgi, A. (Ed.). (1985*). Phenomenology and psychological research.* Pittsburgh, PA: Duquesne University Press.

Giorgi, A. (1992). The idea of human science. *The Humanistic Psychologist, 20* (2, 3), 181-202.

Giorgi, A. (2001). The search for psyche: A human science perspective. In K. J. Schneider, J. T. F. Bugental., & J. F. Pierson, J. (Eds.), *The handbook of humanistic psychology* (pp. 53–64). Thousand Oaks, CA: Sage.

Giorgi, A. (2005). Remaining challenges for humanistic psychology. *Journal of Humanistic Psychology, 45*(2), 204-216.

Gloaguen, V., Cottraux, J. K., Cuchert, M., & Blackburn, I. M. (1998). A meta-analysis of the effects of cognitive therapy in depressed patients. *Journal of Affective Disorders, 49,* 59-72.

Goble, F. G. (1978). *The third force. The psychology of Abraham Maslow.* New York: Grossman.

Goldfried, M. R. (1980). Toward the delineation of therapeutic change principles. *American Psychologist, 35,* 9911-9999.

Gordon, T. (1970). *Parent effectiveness training.* New York: Peter H. Wyden.

Greenberg, L. S., Elliott, R., & Lietaer, G. (1994). Research on experiential psychotherapies. In A. E. Bergin & S. L. Garfield (Eds.), *Handbook of psychotherapy and behavior change* (pp. 509-542). New York: Wiley.

Greening, T. & Bohart, A. (2001). Humanistic psychology and positive psychology. *American Psychologist, 56,* 81-82

Grencavage, L. M. & Norcross, J. C. (1990). Where are the commonalities among the therapeutic common factors? *Professional Psychology: Research and Practice, 21,* 372-378.

Grissom, R. J. (1996). The magical number .7 + - .2: Meta-analysis of the probability of superior outcome in comparisons involving therapy, placebo, and control. *Journal of Consulting and Clinical Psychology, 64,* 973-982.

Haggbloom, S., Warnick, R., Jones, V. K., Yarbrough, G. L., Russell, T. M., Borecky, C. M., McGahhey, R., Powell, J. W. Beavers, and Monte, E. (2002). The 100 most eminent psychologists of the 20th century. *Review of General Psychology, 6*(2), 139-152.

Haigh, G. V. (1971). Response to Koch's assumptions about group process. *Journal of Humanistic Psychology, 11*(2), 129-132.

Heidegger, M. (1977). The origin of the work of art. In D. F. Krell (Ed.), *Martin Heidegger: Basic Writings* (pp. 143-187). San Francisco, CA: HarperSanFrancisco

Hillman, J. (1996). *The soul's code.* New York, NY: Random House.

Howard, K. I., Kopta, S. M., Krause, M. S., & Orlinsky, D. E. (1986). The dose- effect relationship in psychotherapy. *American Psychologist, 41,* 24-28.

Howard, K. I., Luegar, R. J., Maling, M. S., & Martinovich, Z. (1993). A phase model of psychotherapy outcome: Causal mediation of change. *Journal of Consulting and Clinical Psychology, 61,* 678-685.

Hubble, M.A., Duncan, B. L., Miller, S. D. (Eds.), (1999). *The heart & soul of change.* Washington, DC: American Psychological Association.

James, W. (1982). *The varieties of religious experience.* New York: Penguin Books.

Johnson, H. J., & Gelso, C. J. (1980). The effectiveness of time limits in counseling and psychotherapy: A critical review. *The Counseling Psychologist, 9,* 70-83.

Jones, E. (1953). *The life and work of Sigmund Freud: The formative years and the great discoveries* (Vol. 1). New York: Basic Books.

Joyce, J. (1964). *A portrait of the artist as a young man.* New York: Viking Press.

Jung, C. G. (1912/1956). Symbols of transformation (2nd ed.) *The collected works of C. G. Jung* (Vol. 5). Princeton, NJ: Princeton University Press.

Jung, C. G. (1921/1971). *Psychological types. The collected works of C. G. Jung* (Vol. 6). Princeton, NJ: Princeton University Press.

Jung, C. G. (1933). *Modern man in search of a soul.* New York: Harcourt, Brace, & World.

Jung, C. G. (1961). *Memories, dreams, and reflections.* New York: Pantheon.

Kahn, E. (1984). Heinz Kohut and Carl Rogers: A timely comparison. *American Psychologist, 40,* 893-904.

Kaufmann, W. A. (1950*). Nietzsche: philosopher, psychologist, antichrist.* Princeton, NJ: Princeton University Press.

Kaufmann, W. A. (1956). *Existentialism from Dostoevsky to Sartre* New York: World Publishing Company.

Kilpatrick, W. K. (1985). *The emperor's new clothes: The naked truth about the new psychology.* Westchester, IL: Crossway Books.

Kierkegaard, S. (1941). *The sickness unto death.* Princeton, NJ: Princeton University Press.

Kirschenbaum, H. (2009). *The Life and Work of Carl Rogers.* Alexandria, VA: American Counseling Association.

Kirschenbaum, H. & Henderson, V. (Eds.). (1989). *Carl Rogers: Dialogues.* Boston: Houghton Mifflin.

Kirschenbaum, H., & Jourdan, A (2005). The current status of Carl Rogers and the person-centered approach. *Psychotherapy: Theory, Research, Practice, and Training, 42* (1), 37-51.

Koch, S. (1971). The image of man implicit in encounter group theory. *Journal of Humanistic Psychology, 11*(2), 109-128.

Kohlberg, L. (1976). *The meaning and measurement of moral development.* Worcester, MA: Clark University Press.

Kohut, H. (1971). *The analysis of the self.* New York: International Universities Press.

Kohut, H. (1977). *The restoration of the self.* New York: International Universities Press.

Kohut, H. (1982). Introspection, empathy, and the semi-circle of mental health. *International Journal of Psychoanalysis, 63,* 395-407.

Kohut, H. (1984). *How does analysis cure?* Chicago: University of Chicago Press.

Kohut, H. (1985). *Self psychology and the humanities: Reflections on a new psychoanalytic approach.* New York: W. W. Norton & Company.

Koss, M. P. & Butcher, J. N. (1986). Research on brief psychotherapy. In A. E. Bergin & S. L. Garfield (Eds.), *Handbook of psychotherapy and behavior change* (3rd. ed; pp. 627-670). New York: Wiley.

Koss, M. P., & Shiang, J. (1994). Research on brief therapy. In A. E. Bergin & S. L. Garfield (Eds.), *Handbook of psychotherapy and behavior change* (4th ed.; pp. 664-700). New York: Wiley.

Krippner, S. (2001). Research methodology in the light of postmodernity. In K. J. Schneider, J. F. T. Bugental, & J. Frasier (Eds.), *The handbook of humanistic psychology* (289-304). Thousand Oaks, CA: Sage.

Lafferty, P., Beutler, L. E., & Crago, M. (1991). Differences between more and less effective psychotherapists: A study of select therapist variables. *Journal of Consulting and Clinical Psychology, 57,* 76-80.

Lambert, M. J. (1992). Psychotherapy outcome research: Implications for integrative and eclectic therapists. In J. C. Norcross and M. R. Goldfried (Eds.) *Handbook of Psychotherapy Integration* (pp. 94-129). New York: Basic Books.

Lambert, M. J. & Barley, D. E. (2002). Research summary on the therapeutic relationship and psychotherapy outcome. In J. C. Norcross (Ed.) *Psychotherapy relationships that work* (pp. 17-32). Oxford: Oxford University Press.

Lambert, M. J. & Bergin, A. E. (1994). The effectiveness of psychotherapy. In A. E. Bergin & S. L. Garfield (Eds.), *Handbook of psychotherapy and behavior change* (4th ed., pp. 143-189). New York, NY: Wiley.

Lawrence, D. H. (1977). Healing. In V. De Sola Pinto & F. W. Roberts (Eds.), *D. H. Lawrence: The Complete Poems.* New York: Penguin Books.

Lazarus, A. A. & Zur, O. (Eds.) (2002). *Dual relationships and psychotherapy.* New York, NY: Springer.

Leitner, L. M. & Epting, F. (2001). Constructivist approaches to therapy. In K. J. Schneider, J. F. T. Bugental, & J. Frasier (Eds.), *The handbook of humanistic psychology.* (pp. 421-431). Thousand Oaks, CA: Sage.

Levant, R. F. (2004, June). The empirically-validated treatments movement: A practitioner perspective. *Clinical psychology: Science and practice, 11,* 219-224.

Lieberman, M., Yalom, I., & Miles, M. (1973). *Encounter groups: First facts.* New York: Basic Books.

Lilienfeld, S. O., Lohr, J. M., & Morier, D. (2001). The teaching of courses in the science and pseudoscience of psychology: Useful resources. *Teaching of Psychology, 28,* 182-191

Lipsey, M. W., & Wilson, D. B. (1993). The efficacy of psychological, educational, and behavioral treatment: Confirmation from meta-analysis. *American Psychologist, 48,* 1181-1209.

Lohr, J. M., Fowler, K. A., & Lilienfeld, S. O. (2002).The dissemination and promotion of pseudoscience in clinical psychology: The challenge to legitimate clinical science. *The Clinical Psychologist, 55,* 4-10.

Lorca, F. G. (1992). From the Havana lectures. In R. Bly, J. Hillman, & M. Meade (Eds.), *The Rag and Bone Shop of the Heart.* New York: Harper Perennial.

Luborsky, L., Singer, B., & Luborsky, L. (1975). Comparative studies of psychotherapies: Is it true that "everyone has won and all must have prizes"? *Archives of General Psychiatry, 32,* 995-1008.

Luborsky, L., Chandler, M., Auerbach, A.H., Cohen, J., & Bachrach, H. M. (1971). Factors influencing the outcome of psychotherapy: A review of quantitative research. *Psychological Bulletin, 75,* 145-184.

Maslow, A. H. (1954). *Motivation and personality.* New York: Harper & Row.

Maslow, A. H. (1962). *Toward a psychology of being.* New York: Van Nostrand Reinhold.

Maslow, A. H. (1966). *The psychology of science: A reconnaissance.* New York: Harper & Row.

Maslow, A. H. (1971). *The farther reaches of human nature.* New York: Viking.

Maslow, A. H. (1976). *Religions, values, and peak experiences.* New York: Penguin.

Maslow, A. H. (1998). *Maslow on management.* New York: John Wiley.

May, R. (1958). The origins and significance of the existential movement in Psychology. In R. May, E. Angel, & H.E. Ellenberger (Eds.*) Existence: A New Dimension in Psychiatry and Psychology.* New York: Basic Books.

May, R. (1972). *Man's search for himself.* New York: Dell.

May, R. (1974). *Love and will.* New York: Dell.

May, R. (1980). *Psychology and the human dilemma.* New York: Norton.

May, R. (1983). *The discovery of being.* New York: W. W. Norton.

May, R. (1984). *The courage to create.* New York: Bantam.

May, R. (1985). *My quest for beauty.* Dallas, TX: Saybrook.

May, R., Angel, E., & Ellenberger, H. (Eds.). (1958). *Existence: A new dimension in psychiatry and psychology.* New York: Basic Books.

McCready, K. F. (1986). *The medical metaphor: A better model?* Retrieved from www.heall.com/healingnews/dec/medicalmodel.html.

McFall, R. M. (1996). Manifesto for a science of clinical psychology. *The Clinical Psychologist, 44*, 75-88.

Meltzoff, J., & Kornreich, M. (1970). *Research in psychotherapy.* New York: Atherton.

Messer, S. B. & Wampold, B.E. (2000). Let's face the facts: Common factors are more potent than specific therapy ingredients. *Clinical Psychology Research and Practice, 9*, 21-25.

Miller, I. J. (1994). *What managed care is doing to outpatient mental health: A look behind the veil of secrecy.* Boulder, CO: Boulder Psychotherapists' Press.

Miller, I. J. (1996a). Ethical and liability issues concerning invisible rationing. *Professional Psychology: Research and Practice, 27*, 583-587.

Miller, I. J. (1996b). Managed care is harmful to outpatient mental health: A call for accountability. *Professional Psychology: Research and Practice. 27*, 349-363.

Miller, I. J. (1996c). Time-limited brief therapy has gone too far: The result is invisible rationing. *Professional Psychology: Research and Practice. 27,* 567-576.

Miller, W. R. (Ed.). (1999). *Integrating spirituality into treatment.* Washington, DC: American Psychological Association.

Miller, S. D., Wampold, B. E., & Varhely, K. (2008). Direct comparisons of treatment modalities for youth disorders: A meta-analysis. *Psychotherapy Research, 18,* 5-14.

Milton, J. (2002). *The road to malpsychia: Humanistic psychology and our discontents.* San Francisco: Encounter Books.

Montuori, A. & Purser, R. (2001). Humanistic psychology in the workplace. In Schneider, K. J., Bugental, J. T., & Fraser Pierson, J. (Eds.), *The handbook of humanistic psychology.* (pp. 635-645). Thousand Oaks, CA: Sage.

Norcross, J. C. (Ed.). (2001). Empirically supported therapy relationships: Summary report of the Division 29 task force. *Psychotherapy, 38*(4).

Norcross, J. C. (Ed.). (2002). *Psychotherapy relationships that work.* Oxford: Oxford University Press.

O'Hara, M. (2001). Emancipatory therapeutic practice for a new era: A work of retrieval. In Schneider, K. J., Bugental, J. T., & Fraser Pierson, J. (Eds.), *The handbook of humanistic psychology.* (pp. 473 - 489). Thousand Oaks, CA: Sage.

O'Hara, M. (1996, September – October). Divided we stand. *Family Therapy Networker, 20*(5), 47-53.

O'Hara, M. (1997). Relational empathy: Beyond modernist egocentrism to postmodern holistic contextualism. In A. Bohart & L. Greenberg (Eds.), *Empathy reconsidered* (pp. 295- 320). Washington, DC: American Psychological Association.

Orlinsky, D. E., Grave, K., & Parks, B. K. (1994). Process and outcome in psychotherapy – Noch einmal. In A. E. Bergin & S. L. Garfield (Eds.) *Handbook of psychotherapy and behavior change* (pp. 257-310). New York: Wiley.

Orlinsky, D. E. & Howard, K. I. (1986). Process and outcome in psychotherapy. In A. E. Bergin & S. L. Garfield (Eds.), *Handbook of psychotherapy and behavior change* (3rd ed.). (pp. 311-384). New York: Wiley.

Otto, R. (1961). *The idea of the holy*. New York: Oxford University Press.

Prilleltensky, I. & Nelson, G. (2002). *Doing psychology critically: Making a difference in diverse settings*. New York: Palgrave-Macmillan.

Psychotherapy Networker (March/April, 2007). The top 10: The most influential therapists of the past quarter-century (On-line), Available: http://www.psychotherapynetworker.org Retrieved August 19, 2008

Rachman, S. J. & Wilson, G. T. (1980). *The effects of psychological therapy* (2nd ed.). New York: Pergamon Press.

Rennie, E. L. (1990). Toward a representation of the client's experience of the psychotherapy hour. In G. Lietaer, J. Rom bauts, & R. Van Balen (Eds.), *Client-centered and experiential therapy in the nineties* (pp. 155-172). Leuven, Belgium: Leuven University Press.

Rennie, D. L. (1994). Storytelling in psychotherapy: The client's subjective experience. *Psychotherapy, 31*, 234-243.

Rennie, D. L. (1997, April). *Aspects of the client's control of the therapeutic process*. In "The Client's Active Role in Change: Implications for Integration," Symposium at the convention of the Society for the Exploration of Psychotherapy Integration, Toronto, Ontario, Canada.

Resnick, S., Warmoth, A., & Serlin, I. A. (2001). The humanistic psychology and positive psychology connection: Implications for psychotherapy. *Journal of Humanistic Psychology, 41*(1), 73-101.

Rilke, R. M. (1989). Sonnets to Orpheus, II, 29. In S. Mitchell (Ed.), *The Selected Poetry of Rainer Maria Rilke*. New York: Vintage Books.

Robinson, L. A., Berman, J. S., & Neimeyer, R. A. (1990). Psychotherapy for the treatment of depression: A comprehensive review of controlled outcome research. *Psychological Bulletin, 108*, 30-49.

Rosenzweig, S. (1936). Some implicit common factors in diverse methods of psychotherapy: "At last the Dodo said, 'Everyone has won and all must have prizes.'" *American Journal of Orthopsychiatry, 6*, 412-415.

Richards, P.S. & Bergin, A. E. (1997) *A spiritual strategy for counseling and psychotherapy.* Washington, DC: American Psychological Association.

Richards, P. S., Hardman, R. K., & Berrett, M. E. (2007). *Spiritual approaches in the treatment of women with eating disorders.* Washington, DC: American Psychological Association.

Rogers, C. R. (1942). *Counseling and psychotherapy: Newer concepts in practice.* Boston, MA: Houghton-Mifflin.

Rogers, C. R. (1951). *Client-centered therapy.* Boston, MA: Houghton Mifflin.

Rogers, C. R. (1957). The necessary and sufficient conditions of therapeutic personality change. *Journal of Consultative Psychology, 21,* 95-103.

Rogers, C. R. (1959). A theory of therapy, personality and interpersonal relationships as developed in the client-centered framework. In S. Koch (Ed.), *Psychology: A study of a science* (Vol. III: Formulations of the person and the social context). New York: McGraw Hill.

Rogers, C. R. (1961). *On becoming a person: A therapist's view of psychotherapy.* Boston: Houghton Mifflin

Rogers, C. R. (1969). *Freedom to learn: A view of what education might become.* Columbus, OH: Charles Merrill.

Rogers, C. R. (1970). *Carl Rogers on encounter groups.* New York: Harper & Row.

Rogers, C. R. (1977). *Carl Rogers on personal power.* New York: Delacorte Press.

Rogers, C. (1989). Dialogue with Paul Tillich. In H. Kirschenbaum & V. L. Henderson (Eds.), *Carl Rogers: Diaglogues.* Boston, MA: Houghton Mifflin.

Rogers, N. (2008). *Carl Rogers.* Retrieved August 27, 2009, from: http://www.nrogers.com/carlrogers.htm

Rogers, C. R., Gendlin, E. T., Kieseler, D. J., & Truax, C. B. (Eds.). (1967). *The therapeutic relationship and its impact: A study of psychotherapy with schizophrenics.* Madison, WI: University of Wisconsin Press.

Rosenzweig, S. (1936). Some implicit common factors in diverse methods of psychotherapy: "At last the Dodo said, 'Everyone has won and all must have prizes.'" *American Journal of Orthopsychiatry, 6,* 412-415.

Rumi, J. (1984). Say yes quickly. In J. Mayne & C. Barks (Trans.), *Open Secret: Versions of Rumi.* Putney, VT: Threshold Books.

Rumi, J. (1993). In C. Barks (Trans.), *Birdsong.* Athens, GA: Maypop.

Schneider, K. J. (2004). *Rediscovery of awe.* St. Paul, MN: Paragon House.

Schneider, K. J. (Ed.). (2007). *Existential-integrative psychotherapy: Guideposts to the core of practice.* New York: Routledge.

Schneider, K. J. & May, R. (1995). *The psychology of existence: An integrative, clinical perspective.* San Francisco: McGraw-Hill.

Seligman, M. E. P. (1995). The effectiveness of psychotherapy: The *Consumers Reports* study. *American Psychologist, 50,* 965-974.

Seligman, M. E. P. & Csikszentmihalyi, M. (2000). Positive psychology: An introduction. *American Psychologist, 55,* 5-14.

Seligman, M. E. P. (1995). The effectiveness of psychotherapy: The Consumers Reports study. *American Psychologist, 50,* 965-974.

Shadish, W. R., Navarro, A. M., Matt, G. E., & Phillips, G. (2000). The effects of psychological therapies under clinically representative conditions: A meta-analysis. *Psychological Bulletin, 126,* 512-529.

Shafranske, E.P. (Ed.). (1996*). Religion and the clinical practice of psychology.* Washington DC: American Psychology Association.

Sharpiro, D. A. & Shapiro, D. (1982). Meta-analysis of comparative therapy outcome studies: A replication and refinement. *Psychological Bulletin, 92,* 581-604.

Slife, B. D., Reber, J. S., & Richardson, F. C. (Eds.) (2005). *Critical thinking about psychology: Hidden assumptions and plausible alternatives.* Washington, DC: American Psychological Association.

Smith, D. (1982). Trends in counseling and psychotherapy. *American Psychologist, 37,* 802-809.

Smith, M. B. (1990). Humanistic psychology. *Journal of Humanistic Psychology, 30*(4), 6-21.

Smith, M. L. & Glass, G. V. (1977). Meta-analysis of psychotherapy outcome studies. *American Psychologist, 32,* 752-760.

Smith, M. L., Glass, G. V., & Miller, T. I. (1980). *The benefits of psychotherapy.* Baltimore, MD: Johns Hopkins University Press.

Smith, P. B. (1975). Are there adverse effects of sensitivity training? *Journal of Humanistic Psychology, 15*(2), 29-47.

Stang, A. (April 9, 1969). *The review of the news*, p. 16.

Steenbarger, B. N. (1994). Duration and outcome in psychotherapy: An integrative review. *Professional Psychology: Research and Practice, 25*, 111-119.

Stolorow, R. D. (1976). Psychoanalytic reflections on client-centered therapy in the light of modern conceptions of narcissism. *Psychotherapy: Theory Research and Practice, 13*, 26-29.

Szasz, T. (1974). *The myth of mental illness.* New York, NY: Harper and Row.

Szasz, T. (1978). *The myth of psychotherapy.* Garden City, NJ: Doubleday/Anchor Press.

Tallman, K. & Bohart, A. C. (1999). The client as a common factor: Clients as self-healers. In M.A. Hubble, B. L. Duncan, & S. D. Miller (Eds.), *The heart & soul of change: What works in therapy* (pp. 91-131). Washington, DC: American Psychological Association.

Task Force for the Development of Guidelines for the Provision of Humanistic Psychosocial Services. (1997). Guidelines for the provision of humanistic psychosocial services. *The Humanistic Psychologist, 25*(1), 65-107.

Task Force for the Development of Practice Recommendations for the Provision of Humanistic Psychosocial Services (2004). Recommended principles and practices for the provision of humanistic psychosocial services: Alternative to mandated practice and treatment guidelines. *The Humanistic Psychologist. 32*(1), 3-75.

Task Force on Promotion and Dissemination of Psychological Procedures (1995). Training in and dissemination of empirically validated psychological treatments: Report and recommendations. *The Clinical Psychologist, 48*_(1), 3-23.

Taylor, E. (1999a). An intellectual renaissance of humanistic psychology? *Journal of Humanistic psychology, 39*(2), 7-25.

Taylor, E. (1999b). *Shadow culture: Psychology and spirituality in America.* Washington, DC: Counterpoint.

Taylor, E. I. & Martin, F. (2001). Humanistic psychology at the crossroads. In K. J. Schneider, J. T. F. Bugental., & J. F. Pierson, J. (Eds.), *The handbook of humanistic psychology* (pp. 21 -27). Thousand Oaks, CA: Sage.

Thomas, H. F. (2001). Keeping person-centered education alive in academic settings. In K. J. Schneider, J. T. F. Bugental., & J. F. Pierson, J. (Eds.), *The handbook of humanistic psychology* (pp. 555-565). Thousand Oaks, CA: Sage.

Tillich, P. (1952). *The courage to be.* New Haven, CT: Yale University Press.

Tillich, P. (1987). *The essential Tillich.* New York: Macmillan.

Time Magazine (1968, February 23). Stripping body and mind, 1-2.

Tobin, S. A. (1990). Self psychology as a bridge between existential-humanistic psychology and psychoanalysis. *Journal of Humanistic Psychology, 30*(1), 14 – 63.

Tobin, S. A. (1991). A comparison of psychoanalytic self psychology and Carl Rogers's person-centered therapy. *Journal of Humanistic Psychology, 31*(1). 9 – 33.

Vitz, P. (1977). *Psychology as religion: The cult of self-worship.* Grand Rapids, MI: Eerdman's Publishing Company.

Wadlington, W. (2001). Performative therapy: Postmodernizing humanistic psychology. In K. J. Schneider, J. T. F. Bugental., & J. F. Pierson, J. (Eds.), *The handbook of humanistic psychology* (pp. 491-501). Thousand Oaks, CA: Sage.

Waehler, C.A., Kalodner, C.R., Wampold, B.E., & Lichtenberg, J.W. (2000). Empirically supported treatments (ESTs) in perspective: Implications for counseling psychology training. *The Counseling Psychologist, 29,* 657-672.

Waehler, C. A. & Wampold, B. E. (2000). Empirically supported treatments (ESTs) in perspective: Implications for counseling psychology training. *The Counseling Psychologist, 29,* 657-671.

Wampold, B. E. (1997). Methodological problems in identifying efficacious psychotherapies. *Psychotherapy Research, 7,* 21-43.

Wampold, B. E. (2001). *The great psychotherapy debate: Models, methods, and findings.* Mahwah, NJ: Lawrence Erlbaum Associates.

Wampold, B. E. (2005). Do therapies designated as ESTs for specific disorders produce outcomes superior to non-EST therapies? Not a scintilla of evidence to support ESTs as more effective than other treatments. In J. C. Norcross, L. E. Beutler & R. F. Levant (Eds.), *Evidence-based practices in mental health: Debate and dialogue on the fundamental questions* (pp. 299-308, 317-319). Washington, DC : American Psychological Association.

Wampold, B. E. (2007). Psychotherapy: The humanistic (and effective) treatment. *American Psychologist, 62,* 857-873.

Wampold, B. E., Lichtenberg, J. W., & Waehler, C. A. (2002). Principles of empirically-supported interventions in counseling psychology. *The Counseling Psychologist, 30,* 197-217.

Wampold, B. E., Mondin, G. W., Moody, M., Stich, F., Benson, K., & Ahn, H. (1997). A meta-analysis of outcome studies comparing bona fide psychotherapies: Empirically, "All must have prizes." *Psychological Bulletin, 122,* 203-214.

Warmoth, A. (2001). The Old Saybrook 2 report and the outlook for the future. In K. J. Schneider, J. T. F. Bugental., & J. F. Pierson, J. (Eds.), *The handbook of humanistic psychology* (pp. 649-657). Thousand Oaks, CA: Sage.

Watson, J. B. & Raynor, R. (1920). Conditioned emotional reactions. *Experimental Psychology, 3,* 1-14.

Welch, I. D., Tate, G. A., & Richards, F. (Eds.) (1978). *Humanistic psychology.* Buffalo, NY: Prometheus Books.

Wertz, F. (1998). The role of the humanistic movement in the history of psychology. *Journal of Humanistic Psychology, 38*(1), 42-70.

Wertz, F. (2001). Humanistic psychology and the qualitative research tradition. In K. J. Schneider, J. T. F. Bugental., & J. F. Pierson, J. (Eds.), *The handbook of humanistic psychology* (pp. 649-657). Thousand Oaks, CA: Sage.

Westen, D. & Morrison, K. (2001). A multidimensional meta-analysis of treatments for depression, panic, and generalized anxiety disorder: An empirical examination of the status of empirically supported therapies. *Journal of Counseling and Clinical Psychology, 69*(6), 875-899.

Whitaker, R. (2002). *Mad in America: Bad science, bad medicine, and the enduring mistreatment of the mentally ill.* Cambridge, MA: Perseus Publishing.

Yalom, I. (1980). *Existential psychotherapy.* New York: Basic Books.

Young-Breuhl, E. (1988). *Anna Freud: A biography.* New York: Summit Books.

Index

Other Books by the
University of the Rockies Press
www.rockies.edu

Existential Psychology East-West
Edited by Louis Hoffman, Mark Yang, Francis Kaklauskas, and Albert Chan

Awakening to Aging: Glimpsing the Gifts of Aging
Edited by Myrtle Heery and Gregg Richardson

Words Against the Void: Poems by an Existential Psychologist
By Tom Greening

Brilliant Sanity: Buddhist Approaches to Psychotherapy
Edited by Francis Kaklauskas, Susan Nimanheminda, Louis Hoffman, and MacAndrew Jack

CPSIA information can be obtained at www.ICGtesting.com
Printed in the USA
LVOW03s0338130115

422598LV00023B/998/P

9 780976 463887